A HEALTHY-INSPIRED DESSERT
& SWEETS

Sweet FAVES

No Refined Sugar!

Gluten-Free, Dairy-Free,
Nut-Free, Egg-Free,
Vegan & Paleo options

PATTI JORDANNE

© 2021 by Patti Jordanne.
All rights reserved.

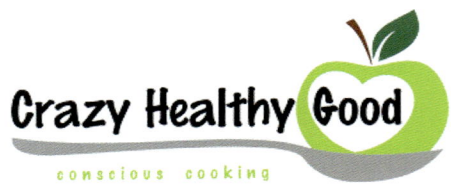

Jordanne, Patti, author
Sweet Faves: Healthy Inspired Sweets & Desserts Cookbook / Patti Jordanne

Includes Recipe Index

Softcover ISBN # 978-1-7773292-0-4

Electronic Book ISBN: 978-1-7773292-1-1
(*available 2022*)

1. Baking   2. Cooking   3. Nutrition   4. Health   5. Cookbooks
6. Refined Sugar-free   7. Gluten-free options   8. Dairy-free options
9. Egg-free options   10. Nut-free options   11. Vegan options   12. Paleo options

Title: Sweet Faves   II. Title: Healthy-Inspired Desserts & Sweets Cookbook

Book Design by Kierra Slater

Photography by Patti Jordanne. All rights reserved.
(*Cover photo: Crunchy Chocolate Bites p.91*)

Printed in Canada
Printed by www.friesens.com

If you're interested in bulk purchases of Sweet Faves for your employees or other premium uses, please contact: sweetfavescookbook@gmail.com

DEDICATION

To Marc, the love of my life.
♥

To Danic, the light in my life.
♥

Bake the world a better place.
♥

CONTENTS

Introduction *5*

Key Ingredients *10*
Baking Tools & Equipment *20*

RECIPES

Bars & Cookies *21*
Cakes & Cupcakes *40*
Desserts, Pies & Tarts *46*
Chocolate *70*
Breakfasts & Beverages *92*
Snacks and "Just for Kids" *103*
Basics *130*

Acknowledgments *150*
Recipe Index *151*

INTRODUCTION

My Story

My Philosophy

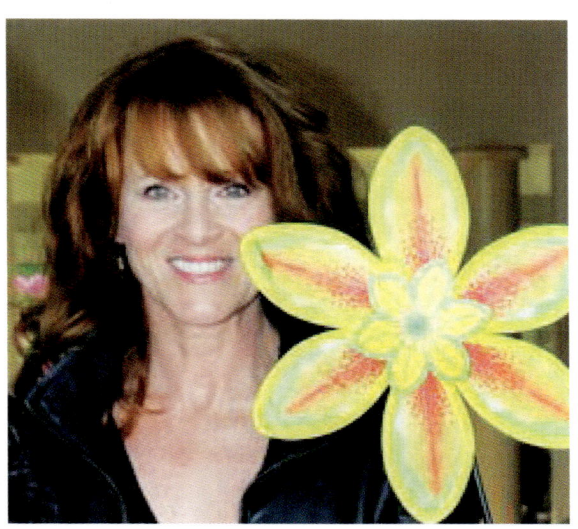

MY STORY

I have been a healthy foodie all my life. However, despite my healthy-eating lifestyle, I still ran in to some health issues. It was a three-year journey of figuring out what was wrong with me! I had a job that I loved for years, but it was very high stress and pressure, with long working hours. That, combined with the necessity to take antibiotics, turned my gastro-intestinal system upside down. Thus began my journey of trying to figure out what was wrong with my gut. Why was I experiencing such abdominal discomfort and IBS symptoms? I was intent on solving the problem, so I immersed myself in education with books, podcasts and online sources, along with regular visits to a variety of healthcare workers—my doctor, acupuncturist, homeopath, naturopath, gastroenterologist, allergist and immunologist. I had too many tests to count and I even had exploratory surgery. Doctors ruled out serious illnesses, which was good, but I still had a gut problem.

During all this, I worked with dieticians, nutritionists and naturopaths. Over the three years I tried various diets: GAPS and SCD, FODMAP, Low Oxalate, SIBO, Raw Food, Candida, Paleo, Vegan, AIP (Auto Immune Protocol) and Ketogenic. As time went on, I was getting worse, so obviously none of these diets were the answer. I also regularly tried cutting out certain foods that might be causing me such pain. I went gluten-free, grain-free, dairy-free, sugar-free, refined foods-free, alcohol-free, sulfite-free, tree nut-free, seeds-free, egg-free, soy-free. I even followed certain diets that required I not eat certain fruits and vegetables. (What the heck?!) At times it felt like I was hardly eating anything—my diet was extremely limited. I lost weight, and I felt worse as time went on. I made my own homemade sauerkraut, kombucha, yogurt and kefir thinking the good bacteria would help. I ate more fat (and made my own homemade, grass-fed ghee), thinking these might heal my gut. All of these diets and diet-limitations were not the answer. It was terrible living with pain and not knowing what the answer was. It was difficult being so limited with what I could eat. I love food and it was hard watching others eat food I couldn't eat!

After three years I finally figured out what the problem was for me. I was allergic to sulfites! And I've since learned that sulfites are an insidious ingredient in a lot of foods. Despite all my life being a healthy cook and eater, this new challenge has forced me to be extra diligent in eating clean, whole foods. I try to stay away from anything that is processed, packaged, canned, or in any way adulterated.

I have always loved sweets, and I have always enjoyed baking. I remember as a teenager spending hours in the kitchen baking cookies, bars, pies and other sweets and desserts so our family could enjoy them for the week of school and work. I remember when I was in university experimenting with healthy food options—not something many university students did. I also remember always experimenting in the kitchen—especially with desserts and sweets.

Because of all my experiences and diets, and because I love food and I love to cook and bake, the result has been a mission to share great recipes that I have created, acquired and adapted, and to share what I've learned by eating healthier. I also want to share the love of good food and the pure enjoyment of eating it! I am now pain free (as long as I stay away from sulfite-containing foods). And the best part is, I have been back in the kitchen creating again, and this time with a wider variety of foods. My favourite things to create are, and always have been, healthy! I am extremely happy knowing I can bake regularly for my family and know that these "treats" are actually good for them and me. **Life is good.**

Please enjoy my collections of baking favourites—hence the book title SWEET FAVES.

MY PHILOSOPHY

I believe in healthy eating. Period. To me, eating healthy means consuming highly nutritious foods that boost my energy and vitality to live a life I wish to live. I think no one diet is the answer for everyone. I borrow from Vegan and Paleo. I borrow from gluten-free, dairy-free and allergy-free for the most part. (I would encourage you to be diligent in determining what diets to borrow from and consider doing your own research to find what is right for you.) Above all else, I believe in eating healthy, organic food as much as I can. I like to eat local, especially getting food directly from the farmers. I like to eat wild fish, organic and pasture raised/grass-fed dairy & meat. I purchase free-range chicken and eggs that provide the most nutrition and are modified the least. I eat healthy fats, organic grains, and organic fruits and vegetables every day. And of course, I indulge in the healthiest desserts and sweets I can drum up! My cookbook expresses the playful way of baking and being healthy while doing it. Please have fun in the kitchen with these recipes—the process can be as enjoyable as the finished product.

MY CHOCOLATE STORY

I am a serious chocolate lover! Years ago, I found that any chocolate that I consumed in the afternoon or evening was enough caffeine to keep me awake at night. But then two things happened: I went to France for a holiday and learned that the farmers in southwest France eat a light breakfast of fresh baguette or croissants with jam. This gives them instant energy to go to work in the fields early in the morning for a few hours before they come back for a big, hearty meal later in the morning. I thought that philosophy also suited me well for my lifestyle since I like to workout in the morning but don't like to eat a lot before my workout. So, then I asked myself: "Why should chocolate be only for dessert?" Chocolate and coffee go really well together, so... I now have my chocolate in the morning with my coffee! It gives me good energy for an hour or so—just enough energy to get me through my workout before I have a hearty breakfast. As a result, I now don't have to worry about the caffeine keeping me awake at night. So that is why, my friends, you can eat chocolate in the morning. Of course, you have to find what works best for you! I do enjoy pure, dark chocolate with my coffee, but many of the chocolate treats in this book are also well-suited for having with your coffee in the morning as a snack or light breakfast, such as Fudgy Butternut Squash Espresso Brownies (p.77), Flourless Chocolate Cake (p.86), or Dark Chocolate Pecan Clusters with Sea Salt (p.87). See the Chocolate chapter! While I do not recommend eating sweets in place of a meal, it can be beneficial to eat sweet foods in moderation, especially if they are filled with nutritious ingredients. Chocolate in its purest form (raw), such as cacao nibs, are rich in antioxidants, so always try to use the darkest chocolate possible. More on chocolate later...

HEALTHY DESSERTS & SWEETS

Healthy Desserts—that sounds like an oxymoron, but it's not. It's time to dispel the myth that all sweets are bad for you. Eating the right sweets in moderation can actually be good for you. Ayurvedic medicine, which has been around for thousands of years, purports that some sweet food in your diet is beneficial for well-rounded and balanced health. There are six "tastes" and sweet is one of them. This is good news for those of us who have a sweet tooth. The trick is to choose sweets that do not contain harmful ingredients, such as refined sugar, high fructose corn syrup, hydrogenated fats, white flour, additives and preservatives. Choose sweets that are full of nutrition, such as high protein, good fats, fibre, vitamins and minerals, antioxidants, etc. Sweets have a bad rap because of all the poor choices that are available. Most of the ingredients I use in this book are chock-full of nutrients! And you can feel good about serving them to your children and your family.

Here are a few examples of nutrient-dense recipes in this cookbook:

RECIPE	POWER INGREDIENTS	NUTRIENTS
Fudgy Butternut Squash Espresso Brownies Page 77	Dates, butternut squash, almonds, raw cacao powder	Dietary fibre, vitamin D, E, B-6, folate, pantothenic acid, manganese, calcium, iron, potassium, phosphorus, protein, magnesium, zinc, riboflavin, copper
Lemon Cashew Cheesecake Page 63	Almonds, coconut, cashews, lemons	Protein, magnesium, riboflavin, calcium, potassium, dietary fibre, vitamin C, E, manganese, zinc, copper, phosphorus, iron, selenium, folate, dietary fibre
Almond Oatmeal Cookies Page 36	Flax seed, oatmeal, almonds, coconut oil	Protein, magnesium, riboflavin, calcium, potassium, dietary fibre, vitamin A, B6, E, K, thiamine, niacin, pantothenic acid, folate, choline, iron, manganese, phosphorus, zinc
Flourless Chocolate Cupcakes Page 45	Quinoa, eggs, raw cacao powder, almond milk, avocado oil	Protein, dietary fibre, vitamin D, calcium, iron, potassium
Queen Elizabeth Date Cake Page 42	Dates, eggs, almonds, walnuts, coconut	Protein, vitamin B6, E, selenium, dietary fibre, calcium, iron, phosphorus, potassium, magnesium, zinc, copper, omega-3, folic acid, manganese
Caramel Pecan Banana Tarts Page 65	Almonds, pecans, almond-butter, bananas, cinnamon	Protein, magnesium, riboflavin, calcium, potassium, dietary fibre, vitamin A, C, E, zinc, phosphorus
Peanut Butter Chocolate Nib'd Truffles Page 73	Peanut butter, cacao nibs, cacao butter	Protein, dietary fibre, phytochemicals, micronutrients, copper, folate, iron, magnesium, manganese, potassium, thiamine, niacin, pantothenic acid, vitamin B6, E, zinc, omega-3, phosphorus, copper
Quinoa Carrot Cake Page 41	Quinoa, coconut, carrots, pineapple, walnuts	Protein, dietary fibre
Berrylicious Cashew Cheesecake Page 49	Pecans, walnuts, dried cranberries, cashews, strawberries, raspberries, blueberries, honey	Protein, dietary fibre, iron, potassium
OMG! Chocolate Avocado Pudding (peanut butter version) Page 85	Avocado, dates, maple syrup, raw cacao powder, coconut milk, peanut butter	Protein, dietary fibre, iron, potassium, calcium
Hazel-Nut-Ella Chocolate Spread (Nutella) Page 144	Hazelnuts, coconut milk, maple syrup, coconut oil	Protein, calcium, iron, potassium, dietary fibre
Parfait Indulgence Page 54	Choices of layers include: fresh fruit, nuts, seeds, buckwheat, coconut, dried fruit, chocolate, avocado, oatmeal	Numerous nutrients, depending on how you build yours

All are rich in antioxidants and contain healthy fats! Adding nutrient-dense foods to your diet is obviously a good idea. However, eating even nutrient-dense desserts and sweets such as these, should be done in moderation. Sweets typically are something you eat once you have already consumed healthy food for the day (such as vegetables and protein)—they are not a substitute for meals.

Above all, have fun baking! The kitchen is a place to play, enjoy the process of creating and serving delights to people you love. Get others involved with you in baking... spouses, friends, children and grandchildren. Be sure to check out the section "Just for Kids"—recipes for kids of all ages! And of course, enjoy eating your tasty creations knowing they are actually good for you.

BAKING WITH KIDS

Children love sweets and they often like to bake. Why not get them interested at a young age in delicious, healthy choices that will help them develop a healthy sweet tooth, and also help them with making healthier choices for a lifetime? In my experience, kids love to "play" in the kitchen. What better way than to have fun with healthy recipes that they can make and eat! I have created a chapter for kids for this very reason. Examples of some easy kids' recipes with NO REFINED SUGAR are:

RECIPE	INGREDIENTS
Apple Chips	Just apples
Banana Soft Serve Ice Cream	Just bananas (with optional add-ins like peanut butter, strawberries or dark chocolate chips)
Blueberry "Instant" Ice Cream	Just coconut milk and blueberries
Power Balls	Peanut butter, rolled oats, sesame seeds, coconut, honey
Fruit on a Stick	Various fruit, dips & toppings
Fudgsicles	Avocados, dates, maple syrup, raw cacao powder, coconut milk

BACK TO BASICS INGREDIENTS

At one point in time, not so long ago, we were made to believe that food that came from packages, containers and cans were not only convenient, but good for you. We have been supporting a multibillion-dollar industry that wants us to believe that processed food is nutritious. The problem is that these conveniences have become part of our health problems in the western world—too much refined sugar, preservatives, sodium, bad fats, chemicals, and additives...among other things. It's time to get back to basics—back to whole foods—foods in their natural state. The recipes in this book do just that. Food has immense power, so the choices we make can greatly affect us. I like to cook and bake from scratch—from ingredients in their natural state. My preference is to purchase certified organic products so I am not ingesting chemicals and hidden additives. (I encourage you to research organic farming practices.) Eating whole foods is better for you, and it's also better for the environment. And eating organic foods is also better for all the workers involved with the growing and harvesting of those foods. Once you have purchased your healthy, sweet pantry ingredients, most of the recipes here are very simple and quick to make. Have a go!

Let food be thy medicine and medicine be thy food.

Even thousands of years ago, Hippocrates, known as "the father of medicine", recognized the importance of eating healthy and using nutritional food to heal.

KEY INGREDIENTS
AND
BAKING TOOLS & EQUIPMENT

Superfoods

Sweeteners & Sugar Substitutes

Staples for a Healthy Sweet Pantry

Allergies & Food Preferences

Baking Tools & Equipment

SUPERFOODS

There are lots of opinions and resources out there on what constitutes a "Superfood". So, what is a Superfood? It is, according to Google, **a nutrient-rich food considered to be especially beneficial for health and well-being.** Many Superfoods are also known for their antioxidant properties. There is no medical definition for Superfoods; it is mainly a current, popular term for food that is extremely nutritious.

What are some examples of so-called Superfoods? This is a list of Superfoods I like to include in my desserts and baking because they pack a powerhouse of nutrition and antioxidants!

1. Quinoa
2. Blueberries
3. Oatmeal
4. Chia Seeds
5. Strawberries
6. Eggs
7. Almonds *(& almond butter & almond flour)*
8. Pistachios
9. Ginger
10. Pumpkins
11. Apples
12. Cranberries
13. Carrots
14. Figs
15. Coconut *(& coconut flour)*
16. Cacao *(pure chocolate)*
17. Buckwheat
18. Hemp Seeds
19. Flaxseeds
20. Pumpkin Seeds
21. Avocados
22. Sweet Potatoes & Yams
23. Cinnamon
24. Healthy Oils *(Extra Virgin Olive, Coconut, Flax, Hemp, Avocado, Cacao Butter)*
25. Butternut Squash
26. Berries
27. Turmeric
28. Honey
29. Walnuts
30. Cashews
31. Goji berries
32. Oranges
33. Gelatin

"No food, including those labelled 'Superfoods', can compensate for unhealthy eating," (Alison Hornby, dietitian, BDA). This concept aligns with my belief that we should be eating healthy every day. Adding so-called Superfoods to your diet is probably a good idea; however, even eating amazing, healthy desserts and sweet treats from recipes provided in this cookbook, need to be consumed in moderation—they are not a substitute for meals. Having said that, there are some treats that would be suitable to be eaten for a quick breakfast: Apple Oat Squares (p.26), Date Squares (p.28), Orange Fig Bars (p.28), Banana Oatmeal Sugar-Free Cookies (p.29), Pecan Rice Crispy Triangles (p.39), Blueberry Crisp (p.55), Pear Crumble (p.59), Lemon Goji Almond Coconut Energy Bars (p.31), or Power Balls (p.109).

Chocolate (as Superfood)
Okay, we all know chocolate is good for us—it really is a Superfood! It's especially nutritious in its most raw form and without added refined sugars. Did you know cacao boosts dopamine and serotonin, which lifts your mood? It also contains anandamide, considered the "bliss molecule"—which makes you feel euphoric. This means eating chocolate can physiologically change your brain to make you feel happier and more motivated. No wonder from ancient times chocolate has been called "Food of the Gods". The Aztecs valued and loved the cacao bean so highly that they used it as currency in their civilization. It packs a powerful punch of antioxidants and minerals. Be sure to get raw cacao powder and not cocoa powder (which is highly processed) for optimal flavour and health benefits. Please note: A few recipes in this cookbook use chocolate chips or baking chocolate. I use good quality, organic chocolate chips (which do contain sugar), but you can purchase chocolate chips made without refined sugar, using instead coconut sugar, stevia or erythritol. You can also use unsweetened chocolate chips or baking chocolate, and then add your own healthy sweetener—an option offered in this book.

SWEETENERS & SUGAR SUBSTITUTES

Research continues to show the harmful effects of consuming refined sugar, such as white and brown sugar, sucrose (glucose & fructose), and high fructose corn syrup (HFCS). Artificial sweeteners like aspartame, sucralose/Splenda, ACE K and saccharin have been known to cause damaging side effects. Fortunately, there are natural sweeteners that are healthy and are tasty alternatives to refined sugars and artificial sweeteners. Pure forms of honey, maple syrup and blackstrap molasses, for example, can actually increase the antioxidant intake in amounts similar to consuming berries and nuts, and provide numerous nutrients like much needed vitamins and minerals. I will explain these and also provide healthy substitutes for sugar.

If I had to narrow it down to just four healthy sweeteners to use in all my baking, I would purchase raw, creamy honey (resource below), pure organic maple syrup, organic coconut sugar and organic dates (medjool or deglet noor).

Best Sweeteners to use: *(Try to use organic when possible)*

Liquid:	Dry:	Fruit:	Vegetables:
- Raw Honey	- Coconut Sugar	- Fresh *(or frozen)* Fruit: bananas, apples, berries, etc.	- Even a few vegetables have been known to sweeten up baking, such as carrots, sweet potatoes, and yams
- Pure Maple Syrup	- Maple Sugar		
- Coconut Nectar	- Lucuma Powder	- Dried Fruit: dates, apricots, cranberries, etc.	
- Blackstrap Molasses	- Date Sugar		
- Balsamic Glaze	- Stevia *(see notes below)*	- Fresh Fruit Preserves: jams, sauces, etc.	
(See notes below about Agave Syrup/Nectar)			

HONEY

A spoonful of honey is veritable liquid gold. Raw honey is a true Superfood and one of my favourite natural sweeteners. Historically honey has been an important part of the human diet. It is packed with enzymes, antioxidants, other proteins, flavonoids, iron, zinc, potassium, calcium, phosphorous, vitamin B6, riboflavin and niacin. Together, these essential nutrients help to neutralize free radicals while promoting the growth of healthy bacteria in the digestive tract. Honey also has antibacterial and antiviral properties. It has also been said that consuming local honey can help with outdoor allergies. Be sure to get honey in its purest form, without added corn syrup, filler or additives. Look for local, raw honey at farmer markets and directly from local beekeepers. The darker the honey, the stronger the flavour; therefore, I tend to use lighter, milder-tasting honey in my baking. Be careful of your source—many companies going for big profits may call their honey organic, natural, pure or grade A, but they may add "cheaper honey" from other countries, or they may even add the dreaded HFCS (corn syrup)! However, they still call it honey. Here is a Canadian resource I buy my honey from. It is creamy and mild flavoured—perfect for baking since it doesn't overpower the flavours in recipes. This honey comes straight from the beekeepers (GC Honey Bees/Grant & Carissa) and it is raw and unpasteurized for maximum health benefits. www.gchoneybees.com

MAPLE SYRUP (pure)

Native to North America, maple syrup is extracted from maple trees. While time consuming, maple syrup processing requires only four steps – drilling the hole in the tree, hanging a bucket to catch the sap, boiling to evaporate out the water, and then filtering of any sediment. Interestingly enough, it takes 45 litres of sap to make 1 litre of maple syrup. Maple syrup is an outstanding source of manganese, and also contains riboflavin, thiamin, calcium, potassium, copper and zinc. Rich with antioxidants, this all-natural sweetener helps to neutralize free radicals and reduce oxidative damage. Scientists have identified more than 67 different plant compounds (or polyphenols)—nine of which are unique to pure maple syrup. Be sure to purchase the purest form of maple syrup (organic, with no added ingredients).

COCONUT NECTAR

Raw Coconut Nectar comes from the sweet sap that is produced from tapping the stalks of stems of the flowering coconut blossom. The watery sap is evaporated at a low temperature to create a pourable syrup. Coconut palms have been traditionally tapped for their sweet nectar for centuries throughout the tropics, especially in the Philippines and parts of Indonesia. I believe coconut nectar is an under-rated sweetener in North America. Not only is it delicious (it doesn't taste like a coconut) and low glycemic, but it is rich in nutrients—vitamin C, potassium, magnesium, zinc, iron and B vitamins. It is rich in other minerals and enzymes, which aid in slow absorption into the blood. Look for raw coconut nectar.

BLACKSTRAP MOLASSES

High in antioxidants and iron. It has a specific flavour that makes it best suited to spiced baked goods such as spiced muffins and ginger cookies. Buy organic to avoid sulfites.

BALSAMIC GLAZE

This is a beautiful sweetener but not often used as a substitute in baking. There are recipes out there using balsamic, such as brownies and strawberry dishes. I have not used balsamic much in baking so I don't refer to it in this cookbook. I do love to use it in savory cooking, however. If you experiment with substituting it as a sweetener in recipes, be aware that it will alter the flavour.

A Note about Agave Syrup/Nectar:
It was not long ago that agave syrup was touted as health food. Juice is extracted from the agave plant, then filtered and heated to break down into a simple sugar called fructose (which is damaging to your health). Agave syrup is a highly refined sweetener that, after the heating and processing, leaves a syrup deficient in nutrients. I would highly recommend choosing the liquid sweeteners I offer above.

COCONUT SUGAR

Most people have heard about the benefits of coconut in its many forms (fresh, milk, water, flour, oil). Now more people are using coconut sugar as their natural sweetener of choice because of its low glycemic load and rich mineral content. In addition, it is easier to digest. It contains polyphenols, iron, zinc calcium, potassium, antioxidants, phosphorous and other phytonutrients. Coconut sugar is extracted sap from the blossoms of the coconut, which is then heated and evaporated to coconut sugar. The process is minimally processed, natural and chemical-free. The beautiful thing is that coconut sugar can be substituted one-to-one for white sugar and brown sugar in most baking. Please note that because coconut sugar doesn't hold as much moisture, it can affect the moisture, texture and consistency of some baked goods.

MAPLE SUGAR

Maple sugar is made from maple syrup. See "Maple Syrup" above for additional information.

LUCUMA POWDER

It is a Superfood fruit from Peru, Ecuador and Chile. Lucuma is known as the "gold of the Incas" and is used to sweeten and flavour desserts and drinks. (It makes a great caramel sauce— see p.131-133) Lucuma can help balance hormones and lower blood pressure. It's rich in beta-carotene, iron, B3, calcium, protein, trace minerals and antioxidants. It is low-glycemic and a good substitution for brown sugar—just use double amount to get the same sweetness.

DATE SUGAR

Date sugar is made from dates. See "Dates" below for additional information.

STEVIA

A great zero-calorie sugar alternative; however, I do not use it in my book because I do not enjoy the taste. Note that not all stevia sweeteners are created equal. There are many different types of stevia—some healthier than others. Keep in mind stevia is 200 times sweeter than sugar, so you don't need much; and because you don't use much, it does not provide any bulk in the baked goods and it will change the outcome.

DATES

Dates are loaded with potassium, copper, iron, manganese, magnesium, vitamin B6 and fibre. From the date palm tree, they are easily digested and help to metabolize proteins, fats and carbohydrates. Evidence shows that dates may help to reduce LDL cholesterol in the blood. Be sure to get organic dates, otherwise, like most dried fruit, they are laced with sulfites. Get soft, organic Medjool dates, if possible. Otherwise, dates such as Deglet Noor are also fine.

OVERCOMING YOUR ADDICTION TO SUGAR

Everyone knows refined sugar is bad for you for many reasons. It is also very addictive and has been likened to the addiction of cocaine. Therefore, I have avoided refined sugar in this cookbook.

SUGAR SUBSTITUTIONS

You can obtain much information online, but here is a simple graph showing substitutions for refined sugar. Please note that all substitutions will have different baking results.

REFINED SUGAR	1 CUP	
Honey	¾ cup	Reduce liquid by ¼ cup
Pure Maple Syrup	¾ cup	Reduce liquid by 3 T.
Coconut Nectar	1 cup	
Blackstrap Molasses	1¼ cups	Reduce liquid by 5 T.
Coconut Sugar	1 cup	
Maple Sugar	¾ - 1 cup	Reduce liquid by 3 T. (but usually not necessary)
Date Sugar	¾ cup	
Lucuma Powder	2 cups	

TIPS FOR OVERCOMING YOUR "SWEET TOOTH"

1. Slowly change to natural, unprocessed types of sweeteners (see above) and start making recipes from this cookbook.
2. Slowly change how much sweetener you put in recipes. (You can often reduce the sweetener by half from traditional dessert recipes.)
3. Use more fruit (and dried fruit) to satisfy your sweet tooth.
4. Believe it or not, adding more fat to your diet will help your sweet tooth to be more satiated (see p.16 for list of healthy fats). Think Ketogenic and Bulletproof philosophies.

STAPLES FOR A HEALTHY SWEET PANTRY

Buy ORGANIC whenever you can! Get local when you can. Definitely buy quality—it makes a difference in the health, taste and texture of your baked goods. Note: weight measuring is more accurate in baking than volume measuring; so, when I give weight measurements, try to weigh those ingredients rather than measuring by volume.

Grains, Flours, Meals, Starches & Cereals
- Spelt Flour
- Gluten-free All-purpose Flour Mix
- Coconut Flour
- Almond Flour *(finely ground blanched almonds)*
- All-Purpose White Flour* *(preferably organic/ unbleached)*
- Quinoa Flour
- Tapioca Flour *(also called starch or powder)*
- Arrowroot Flour *(also called starch or powder)*
- White Rice Flour *(used in 1 recipe)*
- Sorghum Flour
- Cornstarch
- Rolled Oats *(also called Old Fashioned Oats)*
- Quick Oats
- Quinoa
- Millet
- Popcorn Kernels
- Crispy Rice Cereal
- Puffed Quinoa Cereal
- Buckwheat Groats
- Cassava Flour *(optional)*
- Chickpea Flour *(optional)*

Sweeteners
- Honey *(preferably raw, local and mild tasting)*
- Pure Maple Syrup
- Coconut Nectar
- Coconut Sugar
- Maple Sugar
- Blackstrap Molasses
- Lucuma Powder

Fats & Oils
- Coconut Oil *(virgin, unrefined, neutral scent)*
- Butter *(see Dairy section)*
- Ghee *(homemade highly recommended)*
- Avocado Oil *(or other neutral-flavoured oil, such as sunflower or safflower)*
- Cacao Butter
- Coconut Butter
- Coconut Cream *(the solid cream from can of full-fat coconut milk)*
- Olive Oil *(extra virgin)*

Dairy
- Butter, salted & unsalted *(grass-fed and/or organic)*
- Chevre *(used in 1 recipe)*
- Cream Cheese *(used in 2 recipes)*

Extracts *(get pure and quality)*
- Vanilla
- Peppermint
- Orange
- Lemon

Nuts & Seeds** *(raw!)*
- Almonds *(whole & slivered)*
- Cashews
- Pecans
- Walnuts
- Hazelnuts
- Pistachios *(raw or roasted)*
- Macadamia Nuts *(can use roasted)*
- Pumpkin Seeds
- Sunflower Seeds
- Sesame Seeds
- Flax Seeds
- Chia Seeds
- Hemp Seeds/Hearts

Nut Butters
- Almond Butter
- Peanut Butter
- Tahini

(Be sure just nuts—no fillers or added ingredients, except salt.)

Milks
- Coconut Milk*** *(full-fat, canned)*
- Almond Milk *(recipe included)*
- Oat Milk *(recipe included)*
- Cashew Milk *(recipe included)*
- Cashew Cream *(recipe included)*

Spices
- Cinnamon
- Ginger
- Turmeric
- Cardamom
- Nutmeg
- Cloves
- Allspice
- Mace
- Ancho chili powder
- Cayenne

Baking Essentials
- Baking Soda
- Aluminum-free Baking Powder
- Salt: fine sea salt *(Celtic recommended)* & flaked sea salt *(flavoured sea salts optional)*
- Black Pepper

Chocolate**
- Cacao Powder *(pref. raw, organic)*
- Cacao Nibs
- Chocolate Chips *(bittersweet 70-85%)*
- Baking Chocolate *(bittersweet 70- 85%)*
- White Chocolate Chips or Chunks *(used in just 1 recipe)*

Vegetables
- Avocados
- Butternut Squash
- Zucchini
- Carrots
- Ginger Root *(fresh & candied)*
- Fresh Rosemary *(herb)*

Fruit
- Bananas
- Apples
- Berries: raspberries, blueberries, strawberries, blackberries
- Citrus: lemons, limes, oranges, pink grapefruit
- Pears
- Pumpkin Puree *(pure unsweetened in can)*
- Various fruit for Fruit on a Stick & Fruit Dip *(see p.119 & 133)*
- Pineapple Chunks *(unsweetened, canned)*

Dried Fruit
- Coconut *(unsweetened desiccated/fine-shred, long-shred & flaked)*
- Dates *(Medjool and/or Deglet Noor)*
- Figs
- Cranberries
- Goji Berries
- Pineapple
Optional: Mangos, Mulberries, Cherries

Miscellaneous
- Eggs *(large, try to get free-range)*
- Vanilla Beans or Vanilla Bean Powder
- Gelatin Powder *(unflavoured)*
- Espresso *(instant, beans & brewed espresso or coffee)*
- Apple Cider Vinegar *(Bragg's is a good brand)*
- Coconut Butter/Manna
- Quick Cooking Tapioca *(used in 1 recipe)*

WHITE FLOUR*

I try to avoid refined white flour in my baking; however, I have used it 3 or 4 times in this cookbook with recipes that, despite my best efforts, did not convert well to alternative flours. If using, I would recommend to at least get organic, unbleached white (non-GMO), all-purpose flour.

NUTS & SEEDS**

Although it is not necessary, I recommend soaking tree nuts (i.e. cashews, almonds, pecans, walnuts, hazelnuts, pistachios, Brazil nuts) and seeds (i.e. pumpkin, sunflower and sesame) before using. Soaking (and rinsing) removes most of the phytic acid and enzyme inhibitors—both of which are hard to digest. Soaking also results in greater absorption of the many nutrients that nuts offer. I recommend you use organic, raw nuts and seeds for all your purposes. There are some good Canadian companies that sell organic, raw nuts and seeds. Check your sources!

Soak raw nuts and seeds in water for a minimum of two hours. Even better is soaked overnight in a sealed container in the fridge. If you want to learn more, see online resources for ideal soaking times of various nuts and seeds—such as https://fitandfreshlife.com/new-to-raw/what-to-eat/soaking-nuts-chart/.

After soaking nuts or seeds, rinse thoroughly and drain. If you need or want dried nuts or seeds after soaking, simply dehydrate them until they are completely dry. I recommend drying them at a low temperature—at 118° F to maintain nutrients and enzymes.

Once every few months I soak and dehydrate several batches of raw nuts and seeds and keep them in sealed containers in my freezer, ready for use. This may seem like a lot of work, but I only need to do this about once every 3 or 4 months. Storing nuts and seeds in the freezer (whether they are soaked and dehydrated or not) also helps keep them fresher longer, and also keeps rancidity at bay. If you have rancid nuts, throw them out!

If you want roasted nuts, simply roast them after soaking and dehydrating. Roasting brings out a nice flavour for many recipes, such as Dark Chocolate Pecan Clusters with Sea Salt (p.87) and Hazel-Nut-Ella Chocolate Spread (p.144). I don't recommend buying roasted nuts or seeds since they most likely have not been soaked and the shelf life of roasted nuts is often reduced—they often go rancid more quickly.

For added nutrition (and a laborious step), you can even soak and sprout your raw nuts before dehydrating. Find instructions online.

COCONUT MILK***

Get a good quality, organic, full-fat coconut milk. I like Whole Foods 365 brand the best—it contains a good amount of coconut cream and the texture is smooth. Also good are Native Forest and Thai brands.

CHOCOLATE****

I love chocolate, and I also appreciate good-quality chocolate. I like to know the chocolate I buy supports the ethical treatment of the laborers of chocolate around the world. If you possibly can, buy organic, fair trade chocolate.

When melting chocolate, you can use a microwave, but I prefer to control the heat using a bain marie (a water bath). The chocolate is placed in a bowl over a pot of simmering water on the stove. Be sure the bowl does not touch the water. Also be sure the water does not get in to the chocolate or it can cause the chocolate to seize. It is not necessary in this book to temper your chocolate, but there are a couple of recipes I suggest it may be a good idea. Tempering is a method of heating then cooling chocolate so the finished product becomes shiny and hard. If you're interested in tempering, there are many resources online, including video tutorials.

There are lots of ways of making refined sugar-free chocolate. Did you know you could make your own chocolate chips and baking chocolate by buying unsweetened chocolate and sweetening it with a healthy sweetener, such as pure maple syrup, honey or agave nectar? (You can even purchase chocolate chip molds.) Did you know that "raw chocolate" is made using cacao powder (ideally raw, organic), a fat (such as coconut oil, cacao butter, or even butter or ghee) and a healthy sweetener? I include some instructions in various chocolate recipes in this cookbook. However, if you're interested in making your own refined sugar-free chocolate, I would recommend searching online resources.

ALLERGIES & FOOD PREFERENCES

All recipes in this cookbook are refined sugar-free* and soy-free. If you choose organic, most food items will be sulfite-free, so this depends on your shopping choices.

Top allergens in baking are gluten, dairy, eggs and tree nuts. Note that coconut is considered a fruit, seed and nut! People who are allergic to tree nuts may also have an allergy to coconut; however, I do not count coconut as a nut in this cookbook. I include peanuts with all other nuts when nut-free (NF) is indicated.

Following is a list of high allergen foods and diet preferences that I indicate in this cookbook with symbols:

ALLERGEN	SYMBOL
Gluten-free	GF
Dairy-free	DF
Nut-free	NF
Egg-free	EF
DIET-FRIENDLY	**SYMBOL**
Vegan	V
Paleo (grain-free)	P

*Please note: There is one exception to refined sugar-free in this cookbook: A few recipes contain chocolate chips, which most often contain refined sugar. You can now, however, buy chocolate that is sweetened with stevia and/or erythritol. I also offer a refined sugar-free option by using unsweetened chocolate (and adding a healthy/unrefined sweetener) in many of my chocolate recipes.

BAKING TOOLS & EQUIPMENT

The Essentials
Food Processor (fit with S-blade)
High-Speed Blender
Stand Mixer or Electric Hand Mixer
Baking Trays
Muffin Pans (regular size & mini)
Regular & mini muffin liners (silicone or paper)
Pie Pan
Removable Bottom Tart Pans (also called flan pans) (one 9" and six 3")
Springform Pan (approx. 9")
Cake Pans (8x8" and 9x13")
Measuring Cups & Spoons
Cooling Racks
Parchment Paper
Saucepans
Knives
Box Grater
Spatulas
Nut Milk Bag

Optional Items
Digital Kitchen Scale
Microplane Grater
Dehydrator
Immersion Blender or Latté/Milk Frother

Please note:
I mostly use a convection oven when I bake. If you don't have a convection setting on your oven, then you may need to add 10-25% to your baking times.

BARS & COOKIES

Pistachio Lime Squares *23*

Peanut Butter Swirl Protein Bars *25*

Apple Oat Squares *26*

Maple Shortbread *27*

Creamy Coconut Superfood Cookies *27*

Date Squares *28*

Orange Fig Bars *28*

Banana Oatmeal Sugar-Free Cookies *29*

Lemon Goji Almond Coconut Energy Bars *31*

Maple Pecan Bars *31*

Chocolate, Oats & Coconut No-Bake Drop Cookies *32*

Almond Shortbread Fingers *33*

Grandad's Oatmeal Cookies *35*

Almond Oatmeal Cookies *36*

White Chocolate & Macadamia Tahini Cookies *37*

Pecan Rice Crispy Triangles *39*

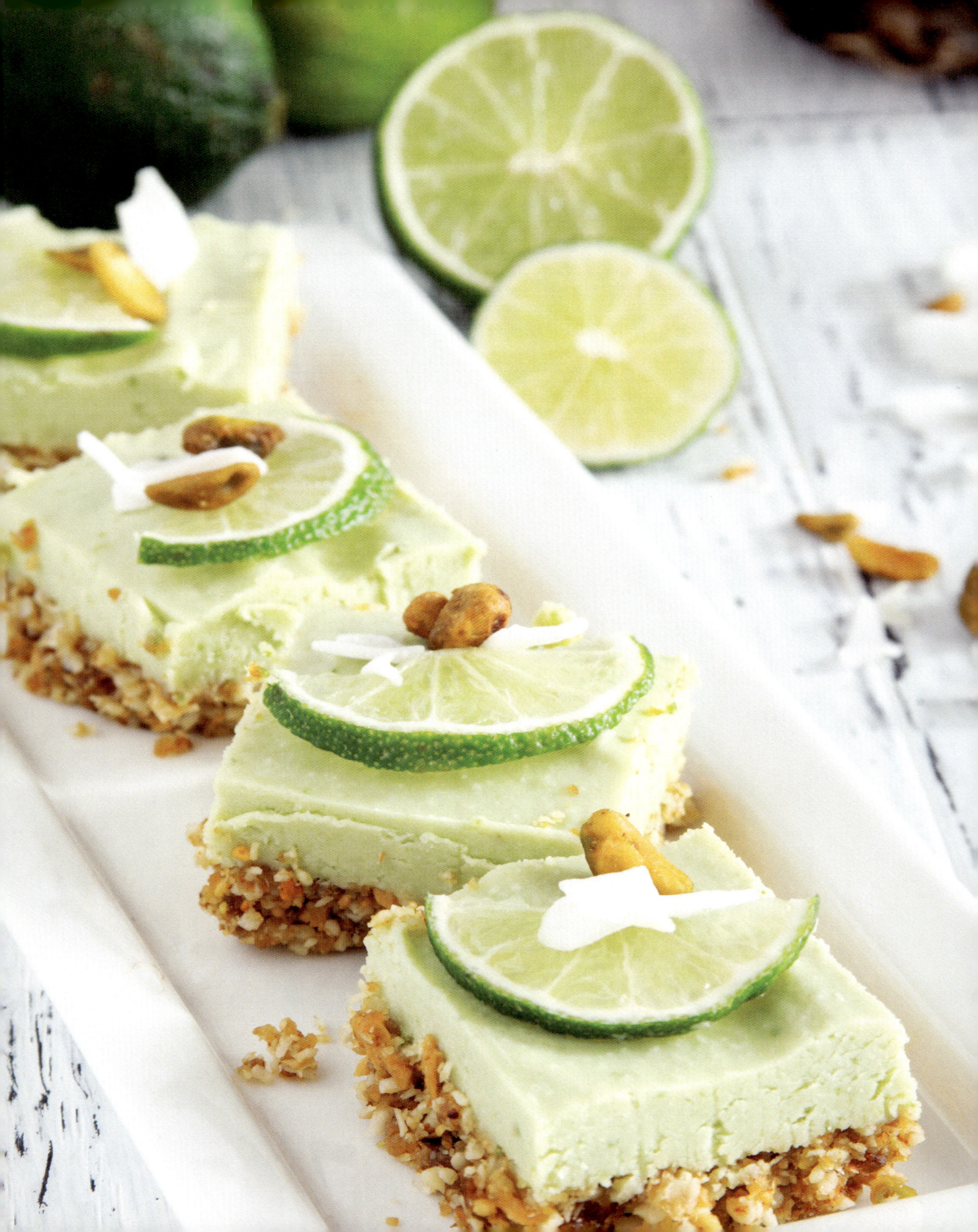

Pistachio LIME SQUARES

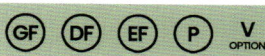

Tangy, tropical and refreshing. Delicious served with Mango Sauce, if desired. These easy, no-bake squares are a good make-ahead dessert. Avocado is the main ingredient of the creamy and smooth filling, but no one ever recognizes it! Inspired by "Sweetly Raw Desserts".

Makes 16 squares   Freezing & Refrigeration Time: 4-6 hours

CRUST
1 cup **shelled pistachio kernels**, raw or roasted (see crust Adaptations)
1 cup **unsweetened shredded coconut**
1 cup **chopped dates** (pits removed)
Pinch **sea salt** (don't use if using salted pistachios)
1 T. **hot water**

FILLING
⅓ cup **fresh lime juice** (zest the limes first!)
¾ cup **mashed, ripe avocado** (approx. 2 avocados)
¼ cup **honey** (For V: use coconut nectar or maple syrup)
½ tsp. **pure vanilla extract**
⅓ cup **virgin coconut oil,** melted & cooled
2-3 T. **coconut butter/manna**, softened/melted (see Tips and filling Adaptations)
2 packed tsp. **lime zest**

Optional:
One recipe Mango Sauce - Use recipe for Raspberry Coulis (p.142), substituting mango for raspberries.

CRUST INSTRUCTIONS
1. Line 8x8" pan with 2 strips of parchment so it comes up 1 inch over sides of pan (for easy removal).
2. In good quality food processor fit with an S-blade, grind together the pistachios and coconut until fine. Add dates (and salt, if using) and process until dried fruit is broken down and mixture is crumbly. Add hot water, a little bit at a time until the mixture sticks together when pressed between thumb and fingers.
3. Press mixture firmly into bottom of prepared pan. Save 2 T. for garnish.

FILLING INSTRUCTIONS
1. In a high-speed blender, add lime juice, avocados, honey and vanilla and blend until smooth. Add the oil, coconut butter and lime zest. Blend again until thoroughly mixed and smooth. Pour the filling over the crust and spread evenly. Sprinkle top with saved 2 T. of crust mixture. (See alternative garnish choices below.)
2. Place the squares in the freezer for 2-3 hours and then transfer to the fridge for another 2-3 hours, or until set. Remove from pan and slice into 16. Serve with Mango Sauce, if using.
3. Store in sealed container in fridge for up to a week.

TIPS
• Coconut butter is also called coconut manna. (It is not coconut oil or cacao butter.) It's pureed coconut meat and it's most often found in a jar (check your local health food store). It's solid at room temperature (and helps in firming the filling)—so you can either scrape off what you need and gently melt it with the coconut oil, or slowly heat the jar up in a saucepan of hot water to soften the contents of the entire jar. (Substitution for coconut butter, see filling adaptations below.)

WAYS YOU CAN ADAPT OR ENHANCE THIS RECIPE
• **Crust:** Only if you have to, substitute raw almonds for the pistachios. You can substitute the dates with dried cranberries.
• **Filling:** If you can't acquire coconut butter, substitute with ½ cup pistachios (soak for minimum 2 hours, then rinse well and drain). For sweeter dessert, add extra 1-2 T. of honey.
• **Garnish choices:** chopped pistachios, shredded or flaked coconut, lime slices, coconut whipped cream or lime zest.
• Option to make in a 8" or 9" round springform pan. Cut into pie wedges.

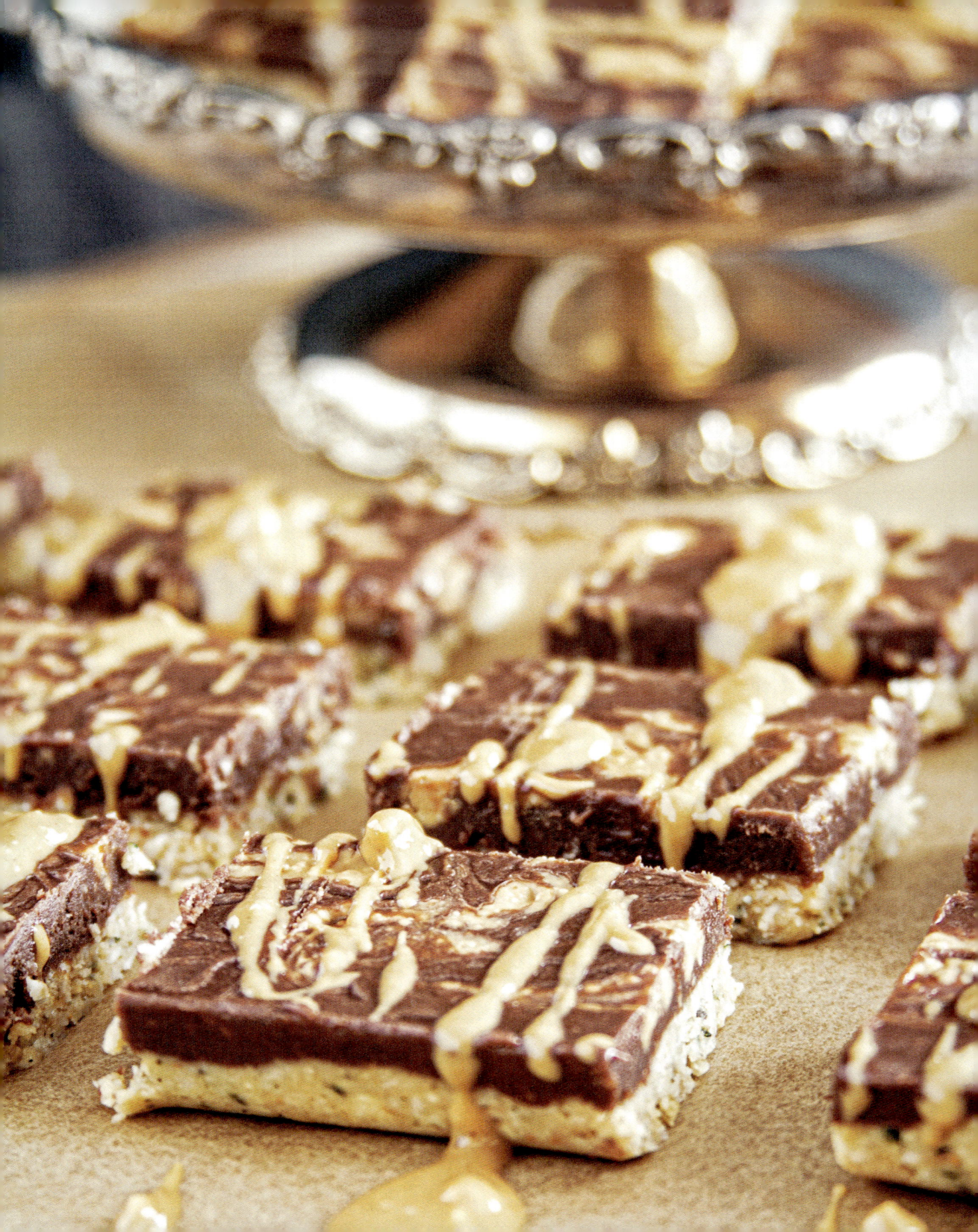

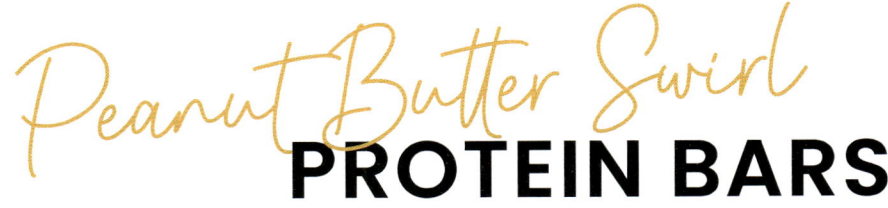
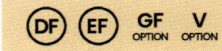

PROTEIN BARS

These no-bake, protein-packed treats contain hemp seeds & peanut butter...a great energy boost at any time of day. And who doesn't like peanut butter and chocolate?!

Makes 16 bars

BOTTOM LAYER
⅓ cup **rolled oats** *(for GF: use gluten-free rolled oats)*
⅓ cup **unsweetened shredded coconut**
½ cup **hemp seeds** *(also called hemp hearts)*
¼ cup **virgin coconut oil**, melted
¼ cup **peanut butter**
2-4 T. **honey,** to taste *(for V: use coconut nectar or pure maple syrup)*

TOP LAYER
¼ cup **virgin coconut oil**, melted
¼ cup **pure maple syrup** *(or honey or coconut nectar)*
3 T. **cacao powder** *(preferably raw, organic)*
3 T. **peanut butter**

FOR SWIRLY PATTERN ON TOP
3-4 T. **peanut butter**, melted

BOTTOM LAYER INSTRUCTIONS
1. In a food processor, blend bottom layer ingredients until mixed evenly.
2. Press firmly into 8X8" pan. Chill in fridge while preparing top layer.

TOP LAYER INSTRUCTIONS
3. In small bowl, whisk together top layer ingredients until smooth.
4. Spread evenly onto chilled bottom layer.

SWIRLY PATTERN INSTRUCTIONS
5. Bring water to boil in a small pot. Place a clean bowl on top of the pot of simmering water. Add peanut butter to bowl, and stir occasionally until melted, about 3-4 minutes.
6. Carefully spoon melted peanut butter in random lines covering the top layer. Use a toothpick to make swirls throughout top layer.
7. Chill in fridge for 2 or more hours before cutting and serving. Store in airtight container in fridge.

WAYS YOU CAN ADAPT OR ENHANCE THIS RECIPE
• Alternatively, if you prefer "cups" instead of bars, press bottom layer mixture firmly into large or small paper-lined muffin cups until each is half full before adding top layer. Add top layer and then make swirly design as described above.

Apple OAT SQUARES

This is a classic Apple Crumble turned in to healthy dessert squares. Need I say more? These are filled with fresh fruit, healthy grains, protein and good fibre. You'll love the apple-cinnamon smell while it's baking!

Makes one 8x8" pan   (Double recipe for 9x13" pan)

EF | GF OPTION | DF OPTION | V OPTION

CRUMB MIXTURE (TOP AND BOTTOM)
1½ cups **rolled oats** *(use gluten-free, if you wish)*
½ cup **almond flour**
½ cup **flour of choice** *(see Tips for flour options)*
¼ tsp. **baking soda**
6 T. **coconut sugar**
6 T. **virgin coconut oil**, melted *(melt together with the butter)*
¾ cup grass-fed butter, melted *(for DF & V: use coconut oil or vegan butter)*

APPLE FILLING
3 cups **cored, quartered and thinly sliced apples** *(see Tips)*
3 T. **coconut sugar** *(or maple sugar)*
1 tsp. **ground cinnamon**

INSTRUCTIONS
1. **Crumb Mixture**: Mix dry ingredients together and add melted oil/butter and mix with fork until course crumbs.
2. Press just over half of mixture firmly into an 8x8" baking pan.
3. **Apple Filling**: In a bowl, mix together apples, maple syrup and cinnamon.
4. **Assembly and Baking**: Place apple mixture on top of crumb mixture. Cover with remaining oat mixture and pat down.
5. Bake 350° F. 40 minutes.
6. Serve warm with vanilla coconut milk ice cream, coconut whipped cream, or Thick Cashew Cream (p.148). Or serve chilled or room temperature.
7. Store at room temperature for 1-2 days.

TIPS:
• Flour options: I like sorghum flour (both sorghum flour & almond flour have protein). Alternately, you can use your favourite gluten-free all-purpose flour mix, spelt flour, organic white unbleached all-purpose flour, oat flour, arrowroot or tapioca flour, or a mixture of these to equal ½ cup. Each flour will result in a slightly different taste and texture. (You can throw in a few finely chopped pecans or walnuts in the crumb mixture, if you like.)
• You can peel apples before slicing, if you like; however, apple peel provides good dietary fibre and nutrients.
• Note that rolled oats from different sources can vary greatly, which can affect the outcome. Try to get rolled oats for this recipe that are not too thick. If your crumble filling falls apart because your rolled oats are thick or coarse, you can use half rolled oats and half quick oats or pulse them a few times in a food processor.

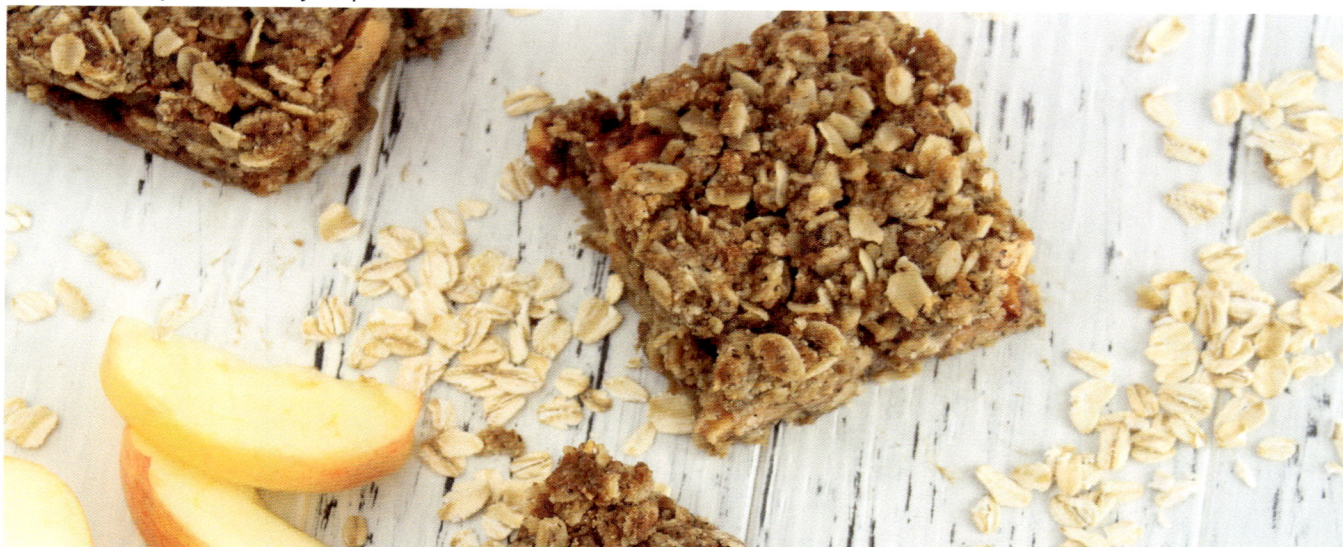

Maple SHORTBREAD

This is an "icebox" or "refrigerator" shortbread cookie. It's very easy to make. Batter is prepared in one bowl. Refrigerate, then slice and bake. This is an old family Christmas recipe (thank you, Dene). We like it so much we stopped making regular shortbread. It is one of only a few recipes in this cookbook in which white, all-purpose flour results in the best outcome.

Makes 24 cookies

INGREDIENTS

1 cup **grass-fed butter**, room temperature *(preferably unsalted)*

½ cup **maple sugar**

1½ cups **spelt flour or white all-purpose flour**, sifted *(see Tips)*

¼ cup **white rice flour**

pinch **sea salt** *(don't need if using salted butter)*

Optional: pecan halves or dried cranberries

INSTRUCTIONS

1. Cream butter until very light. Add maple sugar and beat about 3 minutes.
2. Sift flours and salt. Stir into butter and sugar mixture until just combined.
3. Shape dough into a log about 2" wide and 12" long. Wrap and refrigerate at least 1 hour or overnight.
4. Preheat oven to 300° F. Unwrap and slice into ½" rounds. Arrange on a buttered cookie sheet. Optional: Gently push one pecan half (or dried cranberry) on top of each cookie.
5. Bake 25-30 minutes, until baked through. They should be golden but not brown. Cool on racks. They will crispen up once cool.
6. Store in sealed container in fridge for 3 weeks.

TIPS:

• White flour is traditional in this recipe and often turns out the best product. (I recommend using organic, unbleached flour.) However, I have come to love it made with spelt flour (which does contain gluten)…just be sure to sift the flour after measuring. Unfortunately, I have not found any gluten-free flour mixes that work well in this recipe.

Creamy Coconut SUPERFOOD COOKIES

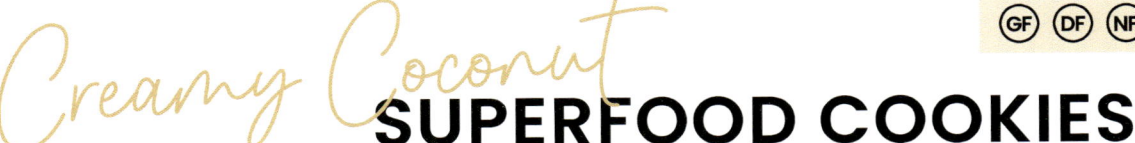

Everyone seems to love these cookies. They are very creamy and satisfying because of the cacao butter and coconut butter—yum! These were created while I was on the GAPS diet to heal my gut. I was craving something sweet so this was the result one day. They are filled with nutrition, protein, healthy fats and several Superfoods! So healthy and delicious, and a great source of energy.

INGREDIENTS

¼ cup *(37g or 1.3 oz.)* **cacao butter**, melted

¾ cup **coconut butter/manna**, softened or melted

3 T. **virgin coconut oil,** melted

½ cup **honey** *(can melt in with coconut oil)*

1½ cups **unsweetened shredded coconut**

1 cup **raw pumpkin seeds**

1 tsp. **vanilla powder**

pinch **sea salt** *(optional)*

INSTRUCTIONS

1. Stir together all ingredients in large bowl. Drop cookies by teaspoon onto a parchment lined baking sheet. Sprinkle with extra coconut, if desired.
2. These will harden at room temperature. They can also be refrigerated to harden faster.
3. Store in fridge or freezer. Good frozen, chilled or room temperature.

TIPS

• Check honey resource on p. 12 for delicious, mild-tasting, creamy raw honey. It's 100% pure Canadian, well-priced, and they deliver.

WAYS YOU CAN ADAPT OR ENHANCE THIS RECIPE

• For V: can substitute honey with coconut nectar or pure maple syrup.
• Optional Additions: 2 T. raw cacao nibs (for more Superfood power!) or ¼ cup chopped, dried cranberries (nice at Christmas time).

Date SQUARES

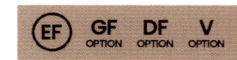

Here in British Columbia we used to call date squares "matrimonial squares". I didn't realize why at the time, I just knew they were good. This healthy adaptation is just as delicious as the original.

Makes 8x8" pan   (Double recipe for 9x13" pan)

CRUMB MIXTURE (TOP AND BOTTOM)

6 T. **coconut sugar**
1½ cups **rolled oats** (for GF: use gluten-free rolled oats)
¼ cup **almond flour**
½ cup **flour of choice** (I use sorghum flour – see Tips for flour options)
¼ tsp. **baking soda**
6 T. **virgin coconut oil**, melted
¼ cup **grass-fed butter**, melted (for GF & V: use more coconut oil)

DATE FILLING

One recipe of **Date Paste** (p.143)

INSTRUCTIONS

1. **Crumb Mixture:** Mix dry ingredients together and add melted oil/butter and mix with fork until coarse crumbs.
2. Press just over half of mixture firmly into an 8x8" baking pan.
3. **Assembly and Baking:** Spread date paste mixture on top of crumb mixture. Cover with remaining oat mixture and pat down.
4. Bake 350° F. 40-45 minutes or until top is lightly browned. Remove from oven and place pan on rack and allow to cool before slicing.
5. Serve warm or room temperature.
6. Store in fridge for up to 5 days.

Orange FIG BARS

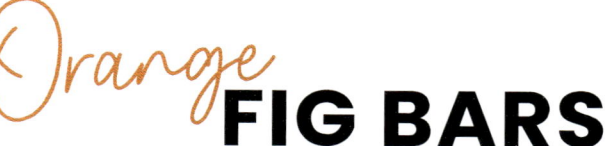
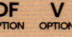

These are like a Fig Newton...but better!

Makes 8x8" pan   (Double recipe for 9x13" pan)

CRUMB MIXTURE (TOP AND BOTTOM)

1 recipe of **Crumb Mixture** (above)

ORANGE FIG LAYER

1½ cups **dried figs**
2 T. **coconut sugar**
1 T. **orange zest**
¼ cup **fresh orange juice**
1 T. **fresh lemon juice**

INSTRUCTIONS

1. Place all Orange Fig layer ingredients in food processor and mix until it becomes a smooth paste.
2. Follow above Date Squares recipe, but use Orange Fig layer between layers of Crumb Mixture.

TIPS

• *Flour options: You can use your favourite gluten-free all-purpose flour mix, spelt flour, organic white unbleached all-purpose flour. If want to use a grain-free flour, such as arrowroot or tapioca flour, then use ¼ cup and increase almond flour to ½ cup. I like sorghum flour—both almond and sorghum flours have protein. Note: Each flour will give you a different flavour, texture and results.*

Banana Oatmeal SUGAR-FREE COOKIES

GF DF NF EF V

Easy, quick, no added sweetener, uber healthy, delicious, and vegan. Banana is used for the sweetener so be sure to use very ripe bananas (ones with lots of brown spots on peel). These are very soft cookies—easy and quick to make in one bowl. They freeze well—just take out 20 minutes before serving.

INGREDIENTS

½ cup **rolled oats** *(for GF: use gluten-free rolled oats)*
1 cup **unsweetened shredded coconut**
1 tsp. **pure vanilla extract**
2 large *(or 3 small)* **very ripe bananas**, mashed
¼ cup **virgin coconut oil**, melted
½ cup **pumpkin seeds** *(or chopped pecans, walnuts or almonds)*
½ tsp. each of **cinnamon, ginger, and cloves**
½ cup **chocolate chips or dried cranberries** *(optional)*
1 flax egg *(see Instructions)*

INSTRUCTIONS

1. To make flax egg, grind 1 T. **flax seeds** in coffee grinder. Mix with 3 T. water; let sit for 10 minutes. (Use as you would an egg in some baking.)
2. Mix together all ingredients well. Form balls and slightly flatten on parchment paper or oiled cookie sheet. (Note—these hold their shape while cooking, so be sure to flatten to desired shape.)
3. Bake 350° F. 20-25 minutes until golden. Cool on wire rack.

Thumbprint Chia Jam Version:

Omit the chocolate chips or dried fruit. Before baking, form a small dent in the middle of each cookie and fill with ½-1 tsp. No-Cook Fruit Jam (p.146).

WAYS YOU CAN ADAPT OR ENHANCE THIS RECIPE

• *Roll each ball in unsweetened shredded coconut before flattening.*

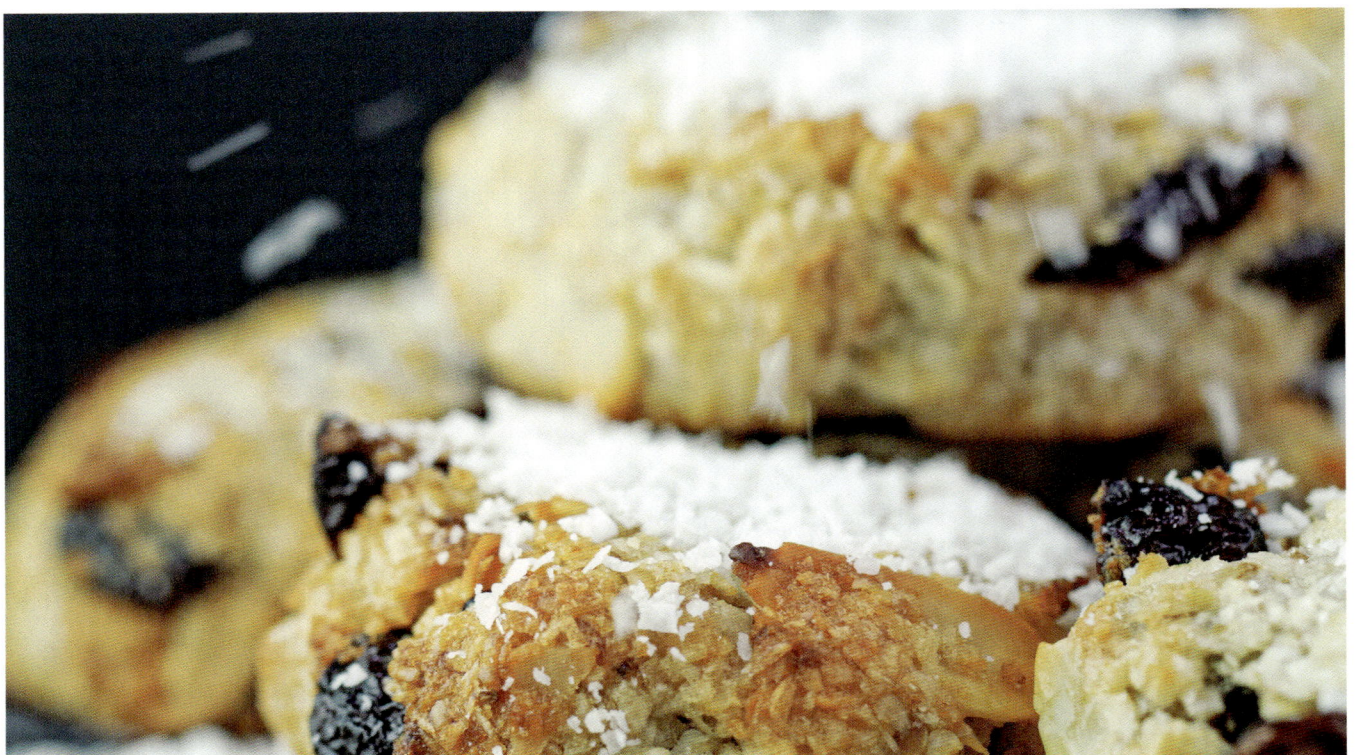

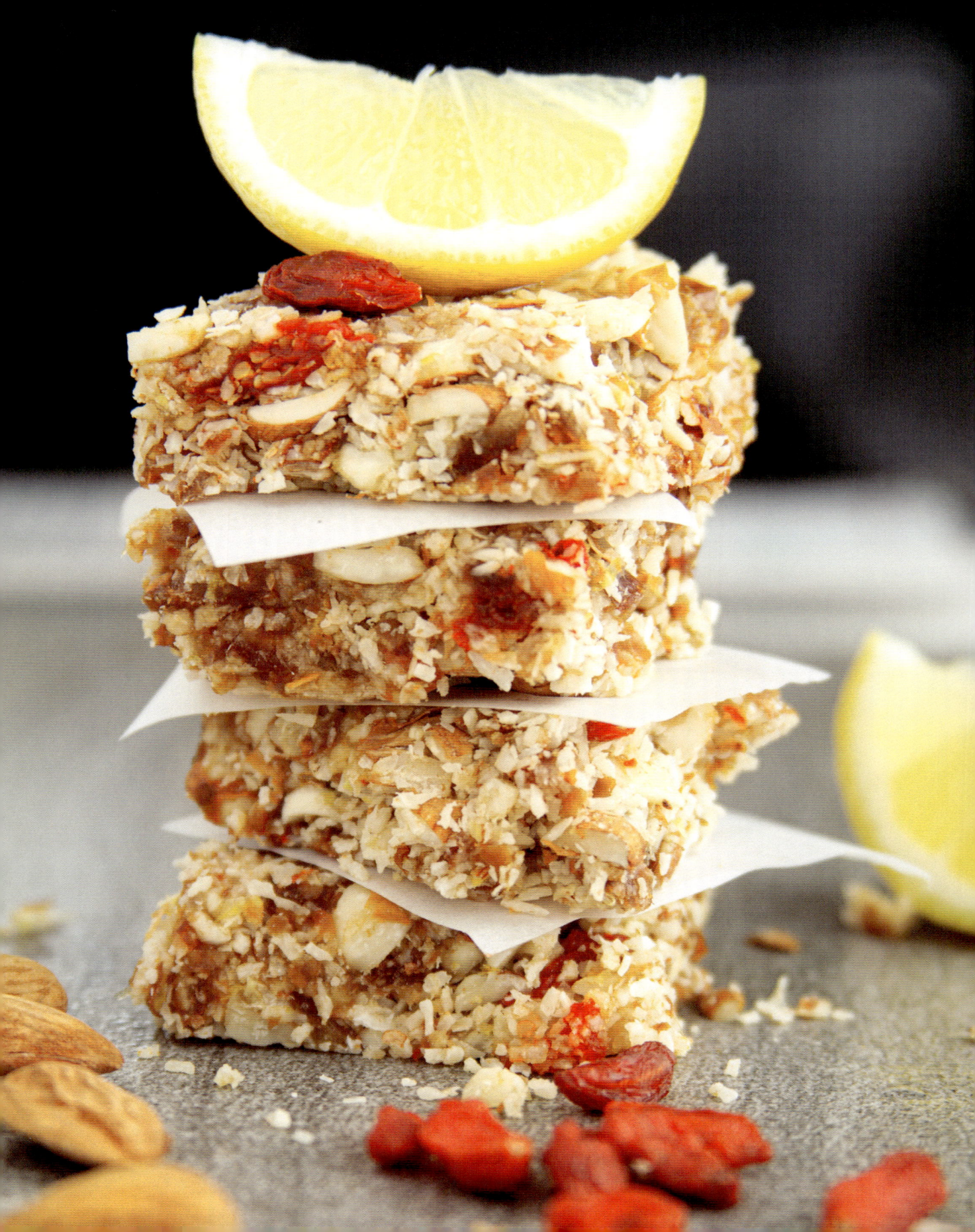

Lemon Goji ALMOND COCONUT ENERGY BARS

GF | DF | EF | V | P | NF OPTION

These are a nice change to typical energy bars made with chocolate and peanut butter. Sweetened only with high energy dates and goji berries, these bars are tangy, tasty and full of protein & energy ingredients.

INGREDIENTS

1½ cups **dates**, pits removed *(medjool or deglet noor)*
1 cup **raw almonds** *(see nut & NF Adaptations below)*
Zest and juice of 1 **lemon**
1 cup **unsweetened shredded coconut**
1 tsp. **pure vanilla**
1 tsp. **sea salt** *(optional)*
¼ cup **goji berries** *(or other dried fruit of your choice)*

INSTRUCTIONS

1. Place the dates in a good quality food processor fit with an S-blade and blend until they're broken down.
2. Then add the rest of the ingredients except the goji berries and pulse until blended but still chunky.
3. Stir in goji berries.
4. Press firmly into 8x8" pan and chill.
5. Cut into bars.

TIPS
- If your dates or goji berries are hard and dried out, soak them in hot water for 5-10 minutes—then drain and pat dry before using.

WAYS YOU CAN ADAPT OR ENHANCE THIS RECIPE
- Feel free to substitute almonds with other nuts. Or for NF: use seeds—such as sunflower, pumpkin or sesame.
- Optional: Add 1 tsp. chia seeds or 1 T. hemp seeds.
- Instead of bars, these can be rolled into balls.

Maple PECAN BARS

A family favourite at Christmas time. (Thanks, Lise.) I've adapted this so it's refined-sugar-free. Tastes like butter tarts and maple pecan pie rolled into one. Yum! I haven't met anyone who doesn't like these!

Makes 8x8" pan   (Double recipe for 9x13" pan)

SHORTBREAD BOTTOM
1 cup **spelt flour or white flour**
2 T. **maple sugar** *(or coconut sugar, ground fine)*
½ cup **grass-fed unsalted butter**, room temperature

TOPPING
⅔ cup **maple sugar** *(or coconut sugar)*
⅓ cup **pure maple syrup**
1 T. **grass-fed unsalted butter**, room temperature
1 **egg**, room temperature
1 tsp. **pure vanilla extract**
¼ tsp. **sea salt**
½ - ⅔ cup **raw pecans**, chopped *(or walnuts)*

TIPS
- If using white flour, try to use organic, unbleached.

INSTRUCTIONS

1. Preheat oven to 350° F. Generously grease 8x8" pan.
2. **Shortbread Bottom:** Mix ingredients in bowl, then press into bottom of prepared pan. Par-bake 25 minutes at 350° F.
3. **Topping:** Meanwhile, mix topping ingredients, except for pecans, in blender or with electric hand mixer.
4. Pour topping on baked shortbread bottom. Sprinkle with pecans. Bake 20-25 minutes more.
5. Cool completely on wire rack, then cut into bars. Serve at room temperature or cold.
6. Store in sealed container in fridge or freezer. (Freezes well.)

Chocolate, Oats, & Coconut
NO-BAKE DROP COOKIES

DF | EF | GF OPTION | V OPTION

These remind me of "Chocolate Drops", a cookie recipe from my childhood. I'm happy to say, this is a much healthier version, and they do taste very similar! This is a fast and easy, no-bake recipe! (Thank you, Susan.) These are good stored in fridge or freezer, so be sure to make a big batch!

Makes 30-40 cookies

INGREDIENTS
- 2½ cups **rolled oats** *(for GF: use GF rolled oats)*
- 1 cup **unsweetened shredded or long-shred coconut**
- ⅔ cup **honey** *(for V: use coconut nectar or pure maple syrup)*
- ½ cup **virgin coconut oil**
- 1 cup **almond butter** *(or peanut butter or any nut or seed butter of choice)*
- 1 T. **whole flax seeds**
- 2 tsp. **pure vanilla extract**
- 6 T. **cacao powder** *(preferably raw, organic)*

INSTRUCTIONS
1. Line a large baking sheet with parchment paper.
2. In a large bowl, mix oats and coconut flakes.
3. In a medium saucepan, combine the honey, coconut oil and almond butter over medium heat and stir continuously until the mixture is melted and mixed evenly. (Do not overheat.)
4. Remove from heat and stir in the oats and coconut mixture.
5. Add flaxseeds, vanilla extract and cacao powder and continue mixing until all is combined.
6. Drop cookies by a tablespoon or small ice cream scoop onto prepared baking sheet. (Optional: Sprinkle each cookie with pinch of flaked sea salt.)
7. Place cookie sheets in the fridge or freezer until they harden.
8. Store in sealed container in fridge or freezer. (If frozen, remove from freezer for 10 minutes before serving.)

TIPS
- Check honey resource on p. 12 for delicious, mild-tasting, creamy raw honey. It's 100% pure Canadian, well-priced, and they deliver.

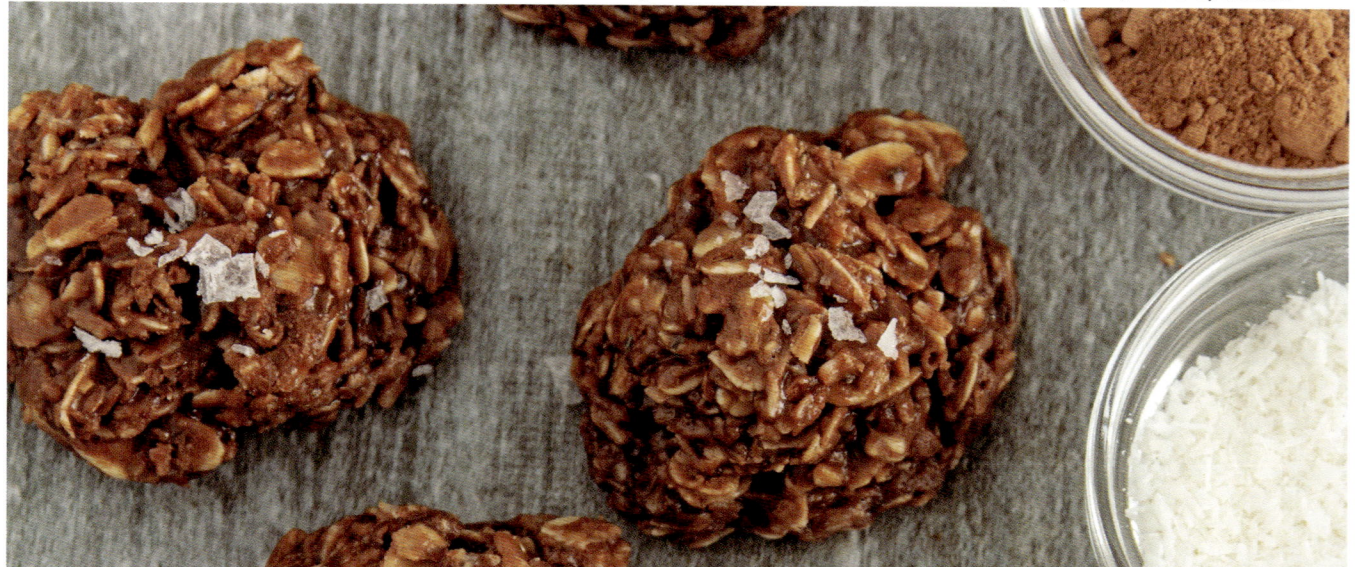

Almond SHORTBREAD FINGERS

This is an old family favorite shortbread cookie. Every Christmas I make this and I get compliments—people seem to like it better than traditional shortbread. I've only adapted it slightly from the original recipe so there is no refined sugar. This can be made gluten-free, but after many tests, I haven't found a gluten-free flour that works well. I have found that white flour consistently produces the best product in taste and texture. My go-to finishing option is #1 below.

Makes 22-26 cookies

INGREDIENTS

1 cup (½ lb.) **grass-fed butter**
¼ cup **coconut sugar** or **maple sugar**, finely ground *(see Tips)*
1 tsp. **pure vanilla extract**
2 cups **organic white all-purpose flour** *(see Adaptations below)*
pinch **salt**
1 tsp. **water**
½ cup **slivered almonds**

Finishing Option 1: ½ cup **maple sugar**, finely ground *(see Tips)*
Finishing Option 2: 1 cup of **dark chocolate**, melted

INSTRUCTIONS

1. In a large bowl, cream butter and sugar for 1-2 minutes with electric mixer or hand beater. Add vanilla and mix for another 30 seconds.
2. Add flour, salt and water. Blend until all ingredients are mixed. Stir in almonds.
3. Roll into finger size lengths.
4. Bake 300° F. for about 45 minutes. (It may take less time. Do not burn.)
5. **Finishing Option 1:** While still hot, roll each finger into sugar and place on cooling rack.
Finishing Option 2: Let cookies cool completely on rack. Melt chocolate and dip half the cookie in and place on parchment paper to set.
6. Store cooled cookies in sealed container in fridge for up to 4 weeks.

TIPS
- To make fine coconut sugar or maple sugar, process in coffee grinder or high-speed blender.

WAYS YOU CAN ADAPT OR ENHANCE THIS RECIPE
- Can substitute white flour with sifted spelt flour.
- Can substitute maple sugar in finishing option #1 with lucuma powder.
- Make into crescent (moon) shape.
- Can use chopped macadamia nuts, pecans or hazelnuts in place of almonds.

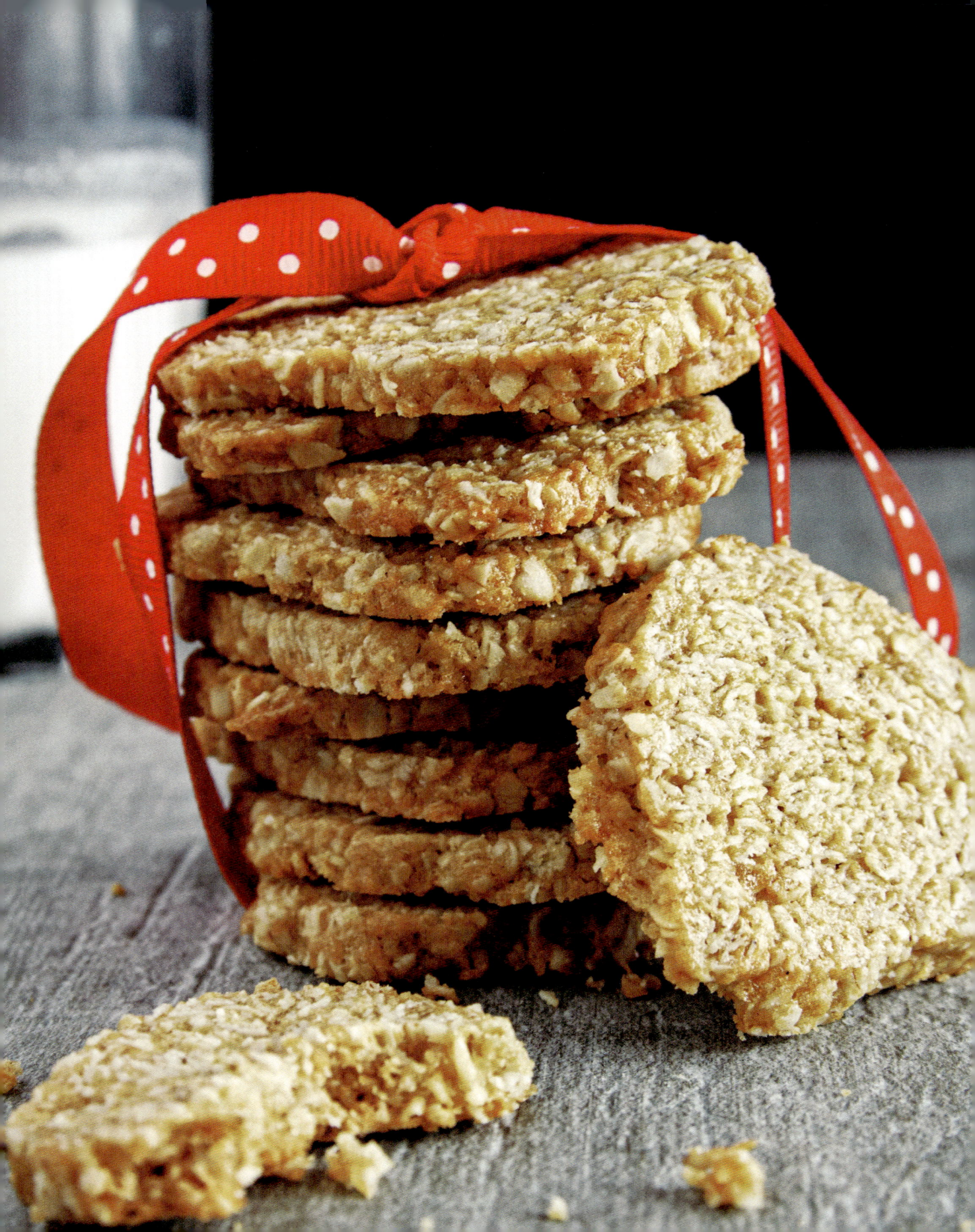

Grandad's OATMEAL COOKIES

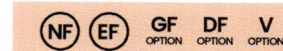

These are a healthy adaptation from an old recipe of my Granny's that she called Grandad's Oatmeal Cookies. My grandparents were born in the late 1800s, so the original recipe has been around for a long time. They still have the same great taste as the original, which thrills me! My grandad would actually spread softened butter on these cookies, and sometimes top with honey. They are easy-to-make cookies (sometimes called ice-box cookies). They are crunchy and delicious and everyone seems to love them. I love having a roll of the raw cookie dough on hand in my freezer so I can easily and quickly slice & bake cookies when people drop by.
(Oh, by the way, the raw dough is delicious, too!)

INGREDIENTS

3 cups **quick oats**
1 cup **white flour** *(or spelt flour) (for GF: see Adaptations below)*
1 cup **coconut sugar** *(or maple sugar)*
pinch **sea salt**
1 cup **grass-fed butter,** melted *(for DF & V: see Adaptations below)*
½ tsp. **baking soda**
¼ cup **boiling water**

INSTRUCTIONS

1. Mix together in large bowl the oats, flour, coconut sugar and salt.
2. Add melted butter and stir.
3. Mix together in a glass measuring cup the baking soda and boiling water.
4. Pour soda/water mixture over the oat mixture and stir well.
5. Divide into 2 parts and roll each into 1½" diameter logs. Wrap tightly in wax paper. Freeze.
6. When frozen, slice logs very thinly. Place on ungreased cookie sheet 1-2" apart and bake in preheated 350° F. oven for about 10 minutes, or until golden.
7. Remove carefully to cooling rack. Let cool until crispy. Delicious warm or cold. Store in sealed container at room temperature or in the fridge for several days.

TIPS
• To make fine coconut sugar or maple sugar, process in coffee grinder or high-speed blender.

WAYS YOU CAN ADAPT OR ENHANCE THIS RECIPE
• Traditionally, these are made with butter, but you must, substitute butter with coconut oil or vegan butter.
• Traditionally, these are made with white flour. Despite many efforts with alternative flours, these cookies turn out the best product using white flour. Be sure to use organic, white unbleached flour. For GF: omit the white or spelt flour and instead use ½ cup sorghum flour and ½ cup arrowroot flour (also called starch or powder).
• The cookies are delicious as is, but you can spread (baked and cooled) cookies with any of the following: soft butter or homemade ghee, honey or Date Paste (p.143). Or mix honey and softened butter (or ghee or coconut oil) together to spread on.

Almond OATMEAL COOKIES

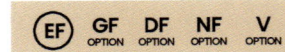

A delicious cookie that is soft on the inside and crunchy on the outside. You'll see what I mean when you make them. I've adapted this recipe from "Oh She Glows". I love these cookies!

Makes 30-40 cookies

INGREDIENTS

2 T. **ground golden flaxseed**
½ cup **virgin coconut oil, grass-fed butter or vegan butter** *(room temperature)*
½ cup **almond butter** *(or other nut or seed butter)*
1 cup **coconut sugar** *(use more or less, depending on your preference)*
2 tsp. **pure vanilla extract**
1 tsp. **baking soda**
1 tsp. **baking powder**
1 tsp. **fine sea salt**
2 cups **rolled oats**, blended into flour *(see Tips)*
(for GF: use gluten-free rolled oats)
2 cups **raw almonds**, blended into almond meal *(see Tips)*

INSTRUCTIONS

1. Preheat the oven to 350° F. Line 2 extra-large baking sheets with parchment paper.
2. In a small bowl, mix together flaxseed and ⅓ cup water. Let sit for 5 minutes to thicken.
3. In a large bowl, beat together the coconut oil (or butter) and the almond butter with a stand or electric hand mixer until well combined.
4. Add coconut sugar and beat for 1 minute.
5. Add flaxseed mixture and vanilla and beat until combined.
6. One at a time, beat in the baking soda, baking powder, salt, oat flour, and almond meal.
7. Fold in the optional additions at this point, if using.
8. Shape dough into 1½" balls, or use a small ice cream scoop, and place on prepared baking sheets, leaving 2 inches between them (they spread out as they bake).
9. Bake 12-15 minutes, until golden brown on bottom. Note: cookies are very soft when they come out of the oven, so let them cool for about 5 minutes before transferring to a cooling rack. Then let them sit for another 10 minutes or so to harden up before eating.
10. Store in sealed container in fridge for up to 2 weeks, or in the freezer for up to 2 months.

TIPS
• Blend rolled oats and almonds (separately) in a food processor (or high-speed blender). I like the flours left coarse-grained, which adds a nice mealy texture to the cookies.

WAYS YOU CAN ADAPT OR ENHANCE THIS RECIPE
• Nut-free option: substitute sunflower butter and sunflower seeds in place of the almond butter and almonds.
• Optional additions: Add ½ cup dark chocolate chips or ½ cup dried cranberries, dried fruit of choice, or finely chopped candied ginger.

White Chocolate & Macadamia TAHINI COOKIES

GF | P | DF OPTION | NF OPTION

These cookies have become a family favourite along with Grandad's Oatmeal Cookies. They are grain-free ...so no flour, no gluten, and no grains (Paleo-friendly). They are super simple and quick to make. And get this—we prefer to eat them when they are frozen. I have offered some substitutions below for the white chocolate and the macadamias...all variations are delicious!

Makes 16-20 cookies

INGREDIENTS

1 cup **tahini** *(250 ml jar, preferably organic)*
½ cup **coconut sugar**
1 large **egg**
2 tsp. **pure vanilla extract**
½ tsp. **baking soda**
¼ tsp. **sea salt** *(optional)*
½ cup good quality **white chocolate chips or chunks**
(see Adaptations below)
½ cup **macadamia nuts**, chopped
(see Adaptations below)

INSTRUCTIONS

1. Preheat oven to 350° F.
2. Line 2 baking sheets with parchment paper.
3. In a large bowl, using an electric hand mixer, combine tahini and coconut sugar. Add egg, vanilla, baking soda and salt. Mix until well blended.
4. Stir in white chocolate and macadamias.
5. Using an ice cream scoop or spoon, scoop out about 2-Tablespoons-sized portions of cookie dough and roll into balls. Leaving about 3 inches of space between cookies, place on cookie sheet. Leave in balls or flatten slightly.
6. Bake 12-14 minutes, or until dry on top and spread. (You may want to rotate your cookie pan half way through baking time for even baking and browning.)
7. Cool cookies on pan for 5 minutes, then transfer to a wire cooling rack until completely cool.
8. Store in sealed container in fridge or freezer.

TIPS

• *Note that when rolling dough into balls, the natural oils from the sesame seeds (tahini) comes out and they seem very oily. This is normal. Remember, all cookies have added fat in the form of oil or butter. When the cookies are baked, however, they don't appear oily... they are moist on the inside and crunchy on the outside. Yum!*
• *This recipe doubles well.*

WAYS YOU CAN ADAPT OR ENHANCE THIS RECIPE

• *This recipe lends itself well to substitute the white chocolate and macadamia nuts with other combinations, such as:*
  • *dried cranberries & pecans*
  • *dark chocolate chips & hazelnuts*
  • *chopped dates & walnuts*
  • *dried apricots & almonds*
  • *dried figs & pistachios.*

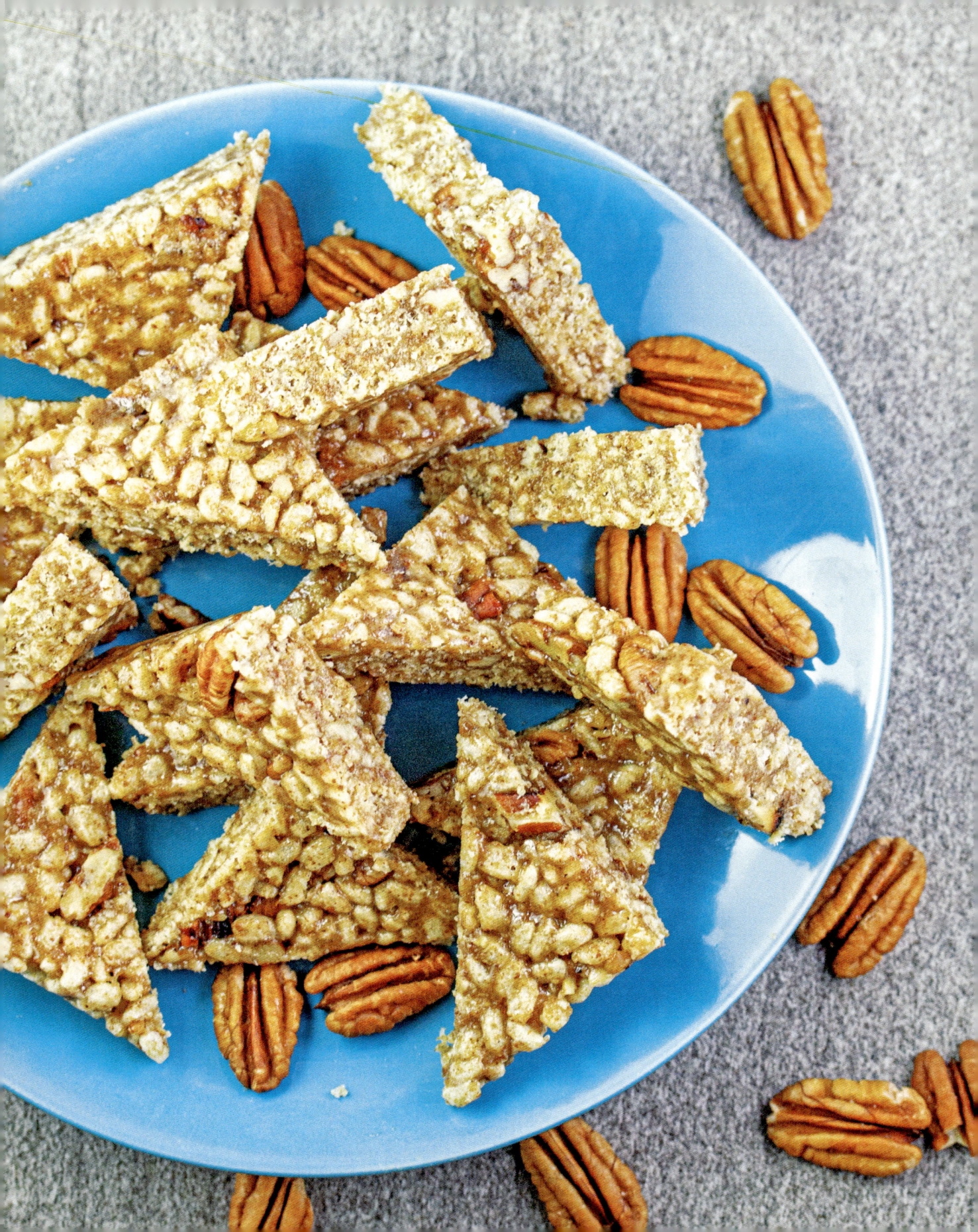

Pecan RICE CRISPY TRIANGLES

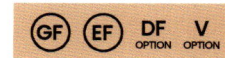

These should be the new Rice Krispie Squares! But these are better—less sweet and much healthier. Okay, it's not a square, it's now a triangle, but that is me being creative. Cut it in squares if you like! Typically rice krispie treats are made with a lot of refined sugar (think marshmallows) and are often too sweet. This is a healthy, yet very tasty, pecan version that is not too sweet and made with organic, crispy rice cereal and unrefined sweetener. The butter or ghee is optional, but I love the flavour of the "butter pecan". These are quick and easy to make and everyone loves them. It's a no-bake recipe with only 5 ingredients (and the option of just 3 ingredients). And yes...they're great for breakfast! HELLO...it's cereal!

Makes 8x8" pan (32 triangles)   (Double recipe for 9x13" pan)

INGREDIENTS

2 ⅔ cup **raw pecans**, divided *(using 2 cups and ⅔ cup separately)*
2 cups **crispy rice cereal** *(I use organic by "Nature's Path")*
⅓ cup **honey** *(for V: use ½ cup coconut nectar)*
1 T. **grass-fed butter** or homemade ghee *(optional)* *(for DF & V: omit)*
2 **pinches sea salt** *(optional)*

INSTRUCTIONS

1. Roast all the pecans in preheated 300° F. oven for 10-12 minutes, or until they are roasted and fragrant. (They burn quickly, so watch carefully.)
2. Divide the roasted nuts: Place 2 cups of the roasted pecans in a food processor (or high-speed blender). Set the other ⅔ cup of pecans aside.
3. Process the 2 cups of pecans until it becomes "pecan butter"—the consistency of nut butter. This may take a few minutes, and you will need to stop occasionally to scrape down the sides.
4. Roughly chop the ⅔ cup roasted pecans and place in large bowl along with crispy rice cereal.
5. In a saucepan, mix together pecan butter, honey and butter or ghee (if using). Warm this mixture very gently. (Do not heat it too much.)
6. Pour warm mixture over rice cereal and roasted, chopped pecans and stir to mix thoroughly.
7. Press mixture firmly into 8x8" pan.
8. Chill in fridge for 10 minutes or longer. Cut into 16 squares, and then again diagonally for triangles. Store in sealed container in fridge for up to 2 weeks.

TIPS
- Making your own nut butter is so easy, you'll wonder why you don't make your own nut butter all the time. You can also make "raw" nut butter...just don't roast the nuts first. Sometimes it's nice to add a little more salt, a pinch of cinnamon, or even a tsp. of coconut sugar or other healthy sweetener. Note: 2 cups of nuts yields 1 cup of nut butter.
- Check honey resource on p. 12 for delicious, mild-tasting, creamy raw honey. It's 100% pure Canadian, well-priced, and they deliver.

WAYS YOU CAN ADAPT OR ENHANCE THIS RECIPE
- You can substitute the pecans in this recipe with your choice of nuts or seeds, such as almonds, hazelnuts or peanuts; however, roasting times will vary. For example, almonds roast for about 10 minutes.
- If you prefer a sweeter version, use an additional 1-2 T. honey.

CAKES & CUPCAKES

Quinoa Carrot Cake *41*

Queen Elizabeth Date Cake *42*
(photo below)

Banana Cake with Crunchy Topping *43*

Blueberry Vanilla Gluten-Free Coffee Cake *44*

Flourless Chocolate Cupcakes with Sugarless Chocolate Frosting *45*

See also:
Chocolate & Chili Quinoa Cake with Chocolate-Chili Ganache *81*
Flourless Chocolate Cake with Raspberry Coulis or Whiskey Caramel Sauce *86*

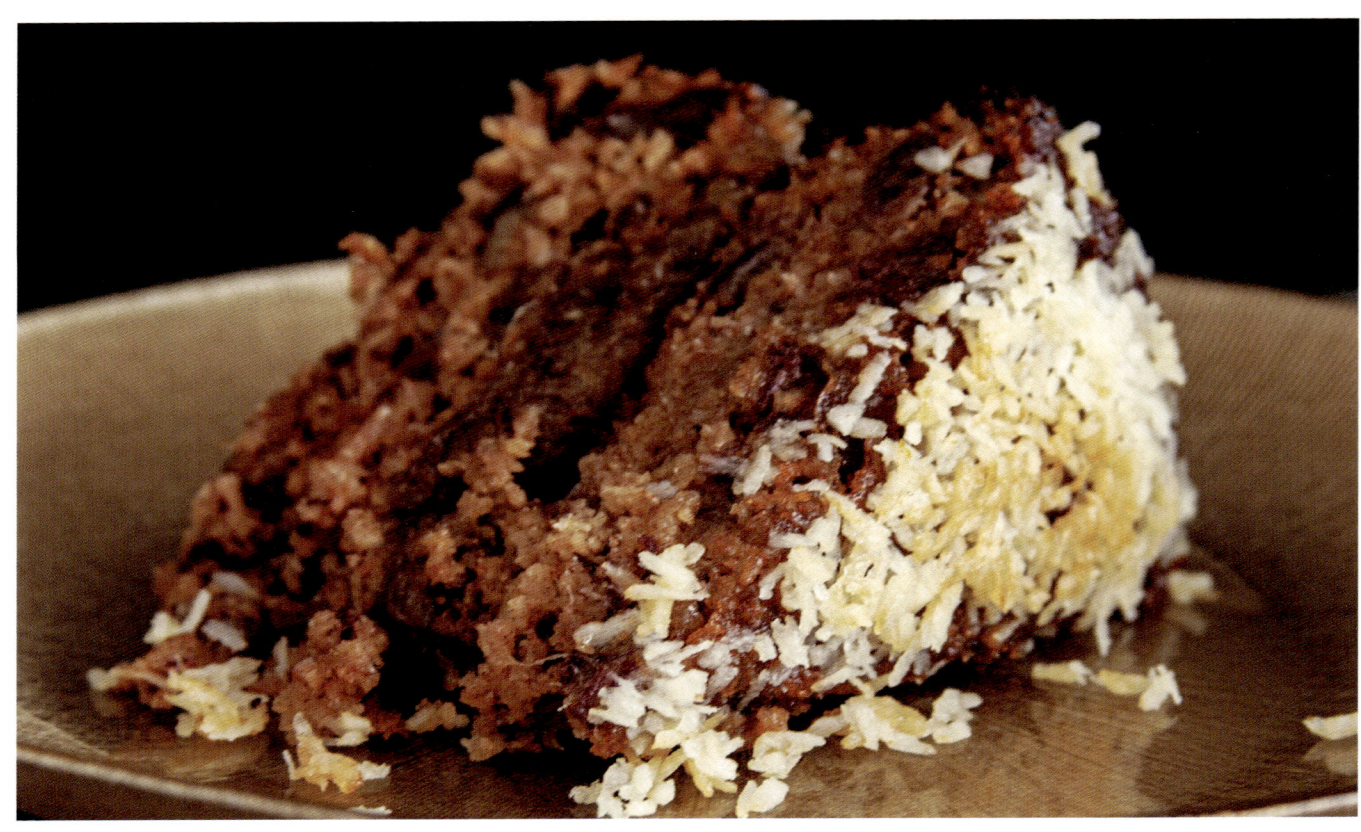

Quinoa CARROT CAKE

GF | **DF OPTION**

This moist and delicious carrot cake is gluten-free, high in protein and nutrients, low in sugar and fat. (The icing is recommended, but optional.) My husband can't get enough of this cake and often eats it for breakfast. This is a feel-good cake! Adapted from "Quinoa 365".

Makes 9x13" cake (or two 8" round cakes)

CAKE

2 cups **quinoa flour**
½ cup **coconut sugar**
3 tsp. **ground cinnamon**
¼ tsp. **nutmeg** *(freshly ground is preferable)*
2 tsp. **baking powder**
2 tsp. **baking soda**
½ tsp. **sea salt**
½ cup **unsweetened shredded coconut**
¾ cup **neutral tasting oil** *(such as avocado or sunflower oil)*
4 **large eggs**
2 tsp. **pure vanilla extract**
3 cups **grated carrots** *(grated finely and packed down)*
2 14-oz. cans well-drained, pureed or finely diced **pineapple** *(save 2 tsp. juice for frosting) (see Tips)*

FROSTING

8 oz. *(250 g)* **cream cheese**, room temperature *(for DF: use DF cream cheese)*
⅓ cup **grass-fed butter**, room temperature *(for DF: use vegan butter)*
2 tsp. saved **pineapple juice** *(or fresh lemon juice)*
½ cup **honey** *(2 T. more if you like sweeter)*
½ cup **raw walnuts** *(or pecans)*, chopped and roasted for 5 minutes in 350° F. oven

INSTRUCTIONS

1. Preheat the oven to 350° F. Generously grease bottom and sides of 9x13" baking pan with coconut oil.
2. **Cake:** In a large bowl, stir together flour, coconut sugar, cinnamon, nutmeg, baking powder, baking soda, salt and coconut.
3. In medium bowl, whisk eggs, oil, and vanilla. Then stir in grated carrots and pineapple.
4. Add the egg-carrot mixture into the flour mixture until all ingredients are just combined.
5. Pour into pan and bake on center rack for about 40 minutes, or until knife inserted in center comes out clean. Place on rack to cool completely before frosting. In the meantime, place cream cheese and butter out to reach room temperature.
6. **Frosting:** In a large bowl, beat cream cheese and butter together with a hand mixer until it's light and fluffy. Add pineapple juice, honey and lemon juice and mix until creamy and smooth.
7. Spread frosting evenly over the top of the cooled cake. Sprinkle with nuts, if you choose.
8. Cut and serve. Cover and refrigerate leftovers for up to 5 days.

TIPS
- You can use fresh or canned pineapple. Roughly puree in small food processor and squeeze out some excess liquid.
- Check honey resource on p. 12 for delicious, mild-tasting, creamy raw honey. It's 100% pure Canadian, well-priced, and they deliver.

WAYS YOU CAN ADAPT OR ENHANCE THIS RECIPE
- If making 2 round cakes, turn it into a layer cake by frosting one cake, then place the second cake on top, then frost the top and sides of the whole cake. You may want to make a double batch of the frosting for this version.
- Decorate top of cake with coconut flakes/ribbons or Honey-Butter Coconut Chips (p.105).

QUEEN ELIZABETH *Date* CAKE

GF | P | DF OPTION

When I was young, my grandmother used to make a cake like this with the same name. It was always a family favourite growing up. I'm not sure if it was the Queen's favourite cake or not, but it is the most delicious, moist and comforting cake I've ever eaten. This recipe is inspired by that cake. I adapted it so there is no white flour or sugar. As a matter of fact, there is no added sweetener at all—the dates naturally sweeten it. It's now my own family's favourite cake. *(Pictured on p.40.)*

Makes 9x13" cake   (Half this recipe for 8x8" cake)

CAKE

500g or 1 lb. *(3-3½ cups)* **dates**, pits removed and chopped finely *(see Tips)*

1½ cups **hot water**

1½ tsp. **baking soda**

½ cup **grass-fed butter**, cut into small cubes
(for DF: use mild tasting oil such as avocado oil)

3 **eggs**, beaten

1 tsp. **pure vanilla extract** *(or ¼ tsp. vanilla powder)*

2 cups **almond flour** or almond meal

1 cup **raw walnuts**, chopped

1 cup **unsweetened shredded coconut**

pinch **sea salt**

ICING

¼ cup **grass-fed butter**, melted
(for DF: use coconut oil or vegan butter)

¼ cup **unsweetened long-shred coconut**

2-3 T. **honey** *(or pure maple syrup or coconut nectar)*

INSTRUCTIONS

1. **Cake:** Generously grease 9x13" baking pan with coconut oil. (Or if using two 8" round pans, grease, then cut parchment paper to line the bottom of pans).
2. In large bowl, pour hot/boiling water over the dates, baking soda and butter. Let mixture cool to room temperature (about 15 minutes). In the meantime, preheat oven to 350° F. and measure out the remaining ingredients.
3. Add remaining ingredients to the bowl and mix with hand or stand mixer until well blended.
4. Pour batter into prepared pan(s) and bake at 350° F. approximately 35-40 minutes, or until done (until toothpick or knife inserted into middle comes out clean).
5. **Icing:** Mix icing ingredients together in small bowl.
6. When cake is finished baking, immediately and carefully spread this icing evenly over top.
7. Place 4 - 6" from broiler and broil icing for 30-60 seconds, until golden, watching carefully it does not burn.
8. Serve cake warm or room temperature.
9. Store covered at room temperature for 3 or 4 days.

TIPS
• You can use any type of dates in this recipe. I like deglet noor because they are easy to work with, less expensive than medjool, and readily available. To avoid sulfites, buy organic. (I prefer medjool dates for a snack, however.)
• Optional: Serve with honey-sweetened yogurt, coconut whipped cream, Thick or Sweetened Cashew Cream (p.148), or crème fraîche and fresh fruit.

WAYS YOU CAN ADAPT OR ENHANCE THIS RECIPE
• This can be made in to a "layer cake" (as pictured on p.40). Simply bake into two 8" round pans and spread the "layer" with Date Paste (p.143), or Thick or Sweetened Cashew Cream (p.148).

BANANA CAKE
with Crunchy Topping

GF | NF | DF OPTION

This cake has been a family staple for many years. And this recipe is the best way to use up ripe bananas. (I often freeze overripe bananas for later use—I just thaw and use.) This cake is moist, delicious, and the topping makes it extra yummy. It certainly does not last long in our house!

Makes 8x8" cake   (Easily doubles for 9x13" cake)

CAKE

¼ cup **milk of choice** *(almond, cashew, oat, cow, etc.)*
¾ tsp. **apple cider vinegar**
1 cup + 1 T. **gluten-free all-purpose flour mix** *(see Tips)*
¾ tsp. **baking powder**
½ tsp. **baking soda**
¼ tsp. **sea salt**
¼ cup **coconut sugar** *(can reduce or omit sugar)*
¼ cup **neutral tasting oil**, such as avocado or sunflower oil
1 cup **mashed overripe bananas** *(approx. 3 bananas) (see Tips)*
1 large **egg**
½ tsp. **pure vanilla extract**

TOPPING

2½ T. **grass-fed butter** *(for DF: use coconut oil or vegan butter)*
¼ cup **coconut sugar**
1 T. **light cream** *(for DF: use coconut cream or Cashew Cream p.148)*
⅓ cup **unsweetened long-shred coconut**
¼ tsp. **pure vanilla**

INSTRUCTIONS

1. Preheat oven to 350° F.
2. Grease 8x8" pan.
3. **Cake:** First make sour milk by combining milk and apple cider vinegar in small measuring cup and let sit 10 minutes. This will be divided into two portions.
4. Combine flour, baking powder, baking soda, salt and coconut sugar in a large bowl.
5. Add oil, mashed bananas, egg, and half of the sour milk to bowl and beat on medium speed for 2 minutes.
6. Then add vanilla and the other half of the sour milk and beat for another minute.
7. Pour into prepared pan. Bake 25 minutes, or until done (toothpick or knife inserted in centre comes out clean). (If doubling recipe for 9x13" cake, bake an additional 5-10 minutes.)
8. While cake is baking, prepare topping.
9. **Topping:** Melt butter in small saucepan. Turn element off and stir in the remaining topping ingredients.
10. Remove cake from oven and immediately spread topping evenly over hot cake. Broil 6" below element for 2-3 minutes letting it bubble for a minute or so until it's golden. Be careful it does not burn.
11. Remove from oven and let cool slightly before serving.
12. Store covered at room temperature 2-3 days.

TIPS
• Not all gluten-free all-purpose flour mixes are created equal. My favourite is Cuisine Soleil Organic GF Flour Mix. Be sure to buy quality—it makes a big difference. I've only tested this recipe with GF all-purpose flour mix, spelt and white flours, and each has their own flavour and texture.
• Bananas should be soft and covered with brown spots. Mash well with fork in shallow bowl, then measure.

WAYS YOU CAN ADAPT OR ENHANCE THIS RECIPE
• Substitute coconut with ¾ cup chopped walnuts or pecans.
• Substitute sour milk with buttermilk.

Blueberry & Vanilla
GLUTEN-FREE COFFEE CAKE

My niece gave me this recipe after I saw her quickly make it after dinner. She whipped it together in no time... and yet it was so, so delicious. And it smells heavenly while it's baking. Who doesn't love healthy & tasty combined with quick & easy?! (Thanks, Trilleen!) Be sure to try the other fruit options—I've tried them in place of the blueberries and they are all delicious!

Makes one 8x8" square cake, an 8" round cake, or 10 cupcakes   (Double recipe to make 9x13" cake)

INGREDIENTS
½ cup **neutral-tasting oil**, such as avocado oil
½ cup **pure maple syrup**
(or honey or coconut nectar)
2 **eggs**, beaten
1½ tsp. **pure vanilla extract** *(I also add a pinch of vanilla powder)*
1 cup **gluten-free all-purpose flour mix**
½ cup **almond meal or almond flour**
1 tsp. **baking powder**
pinch **sea salt**
1¼ cups **fresh or frozen blueberries** *(if using frozen, mostly thaw first)*

INSTRUCTIONS
1. Pre-heat oven to 350° F.
2. Grease 8x8" baking pan.
3. Using a mixer, cream the oil and syrup. Slowly add the eggs and vanilla.
4. Add dry ingredients into wet ingredients and beat until well mixed.
5. Carefully fold in fruit.
6. Spoon into a greased pan and bake at 350° F. for 25-30 minutes or until toothpick comes out clean. (Cupcakes bake about 20-25 minutes.)
7. Good served warm or room temperature.
8. Once completely cooled, cover cake.

TIPS
• Check honey resource on p. 12 for delicious, mild-tasting, creamy raw honey. It's 100% pure Canadian, well-priced, and they deliver.

WAYS YOU CAN ADAPT OR ENHANCE THIS RECIPE
• *Use any of the following: blueberries, raspberries, blackberries, or chopped strawberries, peaches, nectarines or mangos (or a combination of any of these). All are yummy!*

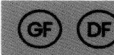

FLOURLESS CHOCOLATE CUPCAKES
with Sugarless Chocolate Frosting

These chocolate treats are made with quinoa and iced with a frosting made with avocado! (And no one seems to know about those 2 healthy ingredients.) Quinoa is a seed, so technically not a grain. These cupcakes are easy to make, are uber moist, have a rich chocolate flavour, and light in texture. They are good on their own—just that much better with the icing. This is chocolate decadence at its best. You feel like you're cheating but these little cakes are good for you! Optional topping suggestions are offered below.

Makes 12 cupcakes

CAKE

⅔ cup **dry quinoa** plus 1⅓ cups **water** *(or 2 cups cooked quinoa)*
¾ cup **neutral-tasting oil** *(I like avocado oil)*
⅓ cup **almond milk**, or milk of choice
4 large **eggs**
1 tsp. **pure vanilla extract**
1 cup **coconut sugar** *(or more, to taste) (or other healthy sweetener)*
1 cup **cacao powder** *(preferably raw, organic)*
1½ tsp. **baking powder**
½ tsp. **baking soda**
½ tsp. **salt**

FROSTING

One batch **Sugarless Chocolate Frosting** (p.136)

INSTRUCTIONS

1. Precook quinoa: Bring water and quinoa to boil in medium saucepan, then reduce to simmer. Cover with a tight-fitting lid, and cook for 12 minutes. Turn heat off, place a piece of paper towel over the saucepan and place the lid back on. Let sit for another 8-10 minutes. Take lid off, fluff with fork, and let cool.
2. Preheat oven to 350° F.
3. Line muffin pan with 12 paper liners (or grease muffin pan).
4. In a blender, combine oil, milk, eggs and vanilla extract and process briefly. Add the cooled, cooked quinoa and blend until smooth and creamy.
5. In a large bowl, whisk together sugar, cocoa powder, b. powder, b. soda, and salt, removing any lumps. Add blender ingredients to bowl of dry ingredients. Whisk or mix with an electric hand mixer until well combined and smooth.
6. Divide batter evenly into the 12 cupcake liners. Bake 25-28 minutes, or until toothpick inserted in center comes out clean.
7. Remove from oven and let pans cool on rack. When cupcakes are completely cool, spread or pipe on Sugarless Chocolate Frosting.
8. Store in sealed container for 2-3 days. Freezes well for up to a month.

WAYS YOU CAN ADAPT OR ENHANCE THIS RECIPE

• After frosting the cupcakes, top with shaved chocolate, Salty, Sweet & Spicy Maple Pecans (p.114), Sprinkles (p.125), or Honey Butter Coconut Chips (p.105). Or drizzle with your favourite Caramel Sauce (p.131-133) and maybe add a pinch of fleur de sel or flaked sea salt.
• You can make this recipe into two 8" round pans for a layer cake by frosting one cake, then place the second cake on top, then frost the top and sides of the whole cake. You may need to make more frosting!

DESSERTS, PIES & TARTS

Apple Tart Pie with Butter Crust *47*

Berrylicious Cashew Cheesecake *49*

Blueberry "Instant" Ice Cream *50*

Baked Coconut Eggnog Custard *51*

Fresh Raspberry Pie with Raspberry-Honey Glaze *53*

Parfait Indulgence *54*

Blueberry Crisp *55*

Lemon & Lime Frozen Mini Cashew Cheesecakes *57*

Pumpkin Spice Custard Cups *58*

Pumpkin Pie *58*

Pear Crumble *59*

Coconut Chia Pudding with Berry Sauce *61*

Lemon Cashew Cheesecake *63*

Maple Syrup Pie *64*

Caramel Pecan Banana Tarts *65*

Lemon Tarts *67*

Baked Cashew Cheesecake with Caramelized Apples *69*

APPLE TART PIE
with Butter Crust

NF | EF | V | GF OPTION | DF OPTION

This is my favourite apple pie. It's actually a tart—no top crust (so less work). The smell of it baking is pure heaven! This is one of those old recipes I've adapted to make it healthier. The butter compliments the taste of the apple and cinnamon, so I recommend you make either the Butter-Vinegar Shortbread Crust or the Spelt & Butter Shortbread Crust. (Don't let the vinegar fool you—you can't taste it and it makes for a tender crust.) However, gluten-free and dairy-free crust options are provided.

Makes one pie-sized tart—use 9" removable bottom tart pan

CRUST
Butter-Vinegar Crust (140)
or Spelt & Butter Shortbread Crust (p.138)
For GF: use Pecan Oat Crust (p.139)
For DF: use Easy Oil Crust (p.137)

APPLE FILLING
3 T. **pure maple syrup**
2 T. **maple sugar** *(or coconut sugar, ground finely)*
2 Tbsp. **flour**—your choice of spelt or white
(for GF: use sorghum, coconut, buckwheat or oat flour
¾ tsp. **cinnamon**
3½ cups **coarsely grated apple** *(see Tips for best apples to use)*

INSTRUCTIONS
1. **Crust:** Prepare crust as per recipe and refrigerate in pan until using. (You can parbake 350° F. for 8 minutes, if you choose.)
2. **Filling:** Mix together apple filling in medium-sized bowl.
3. Spread filling evenly over butter pie crust.
4. Bake approximately 1 hour at 400° F. (Some ovens may need to be turned down to 375° F. to prevent crust from burning, so check during baking. Or use a loose foil "tent" over pie or pie crust.)
5. Remove from oven and cool for 10 minutes or longer.
6. Serve warm or cooled. Optional: serve with maple syrup sweetened coconut whipped cream or Cashew Cream (p.148) and a dusting of cinnamon. Or drizzle Salted Caramel Sauce (p.133) on top of each slice.

TIPS
• You can make your own oat flour by blending rolled oats in a blender or food processor until very fine. You can make your own buckwheat flour by blending buckwheat groats in food processor for about 5 minutes.
• Good baking apples are: Gala, Granny Smith, Fuji, Pink Lady & Honeycrisp.

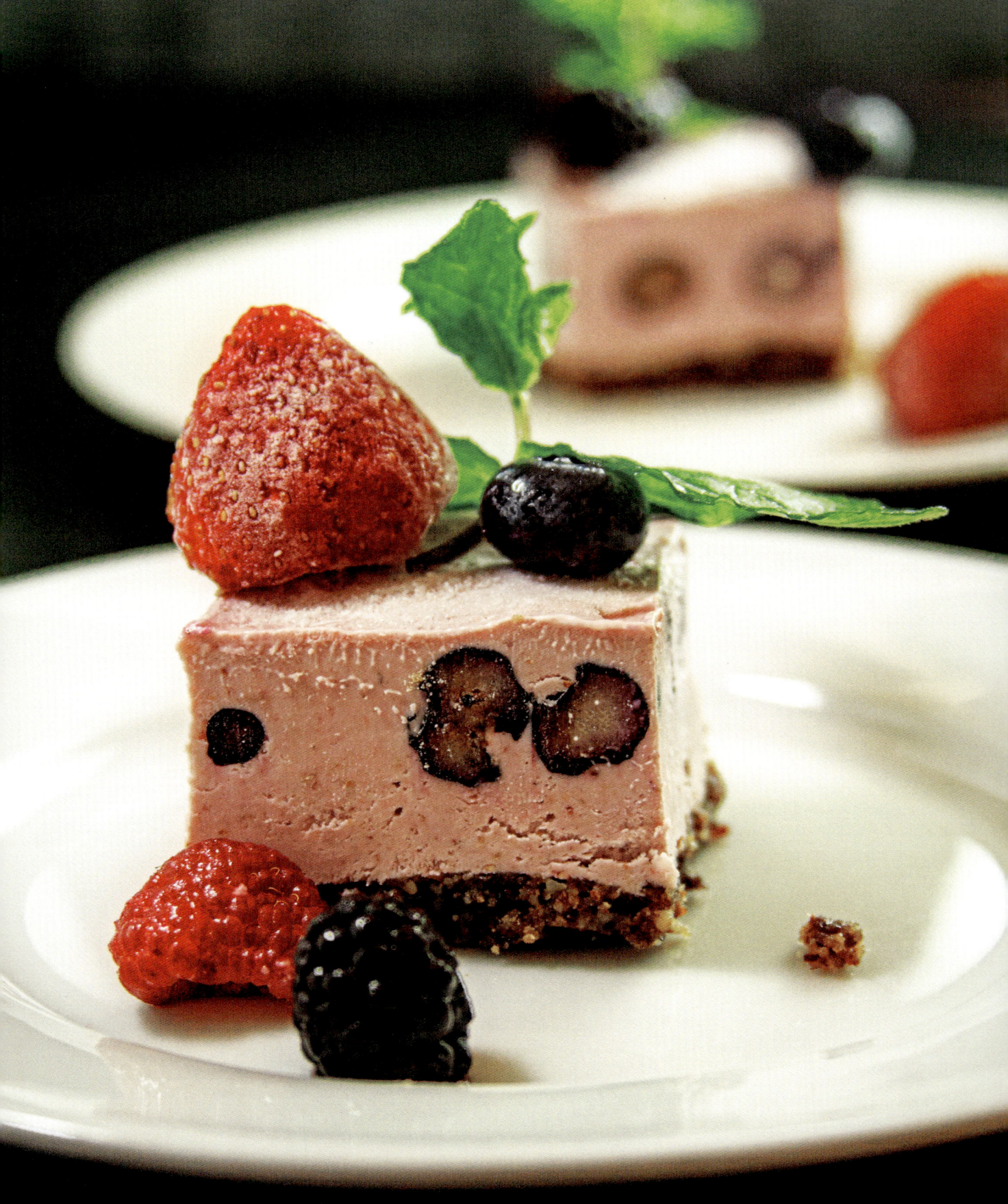

Berrylicious CASHEW CHEESECAKE

GF | DF | EF | P | V OPTION

This is a recipe from my dear friend, Susan. It is an absolutely delicious frozen cheesecake and it's good served in any season. It is impressive to look at, too! You can make a big cheesecake that keeps in the freezer for several weeks, or make into individual cheesecakes.

Serves 10-12: Makes one 8" square pan, one 9" round springform pan, two 5" springform or removable bottom cake pans, or 7-8 mini-cheesecakes
Freezing time: Minimum 4 hours

CRUST
1 cup **raw pecans**
1 cup **raw walnuts**
1 cup **dried cranberries** *(or dried cherries)*
1 T. **hot water**

FILLING
2 cups **raw cashews**, soaked in water for at least 2 hours or overnight in fridge, then rinse and drain
½ cup **virgin coconut oil**, melted
1 T. **fresh lemon juice**
½ cup **honey** *(for V: use pure maple syrup or coconut nectar)*
1 tsp. **pure vanilla extract**
2 cups **fresh or frozen strawberries** *(if frozen, thaw first)*
1 cup **frozen whole raspberries and blueberries** *(approx. ½ cup of each) (keep frozen until use.)*

SERVING INSTRUCTIONS
Remove from freezer about 20 minutes prior to serving. (Be sure to slice cheesecake while still fully frozen—you'll then get a nice cut through the berries.) Remove the cheesecake from the pan onto a cutting board. Cut into pieces and serve as is, or with extra fresh berries on top, coconut whipped cream, sprigs of mint, or a drizzle of Raspberry Coulis (p.142). (Store remaining cheesecake, well wrapped and sealed, in freezer for up to 2 months.)

CRUST INSTRUCTIONS
1. Roast pecans and walnuts on baking sheet at 350°F. for about 7 minutes, or until toasted and fragrant. Let cool a few minutes. (If prefer "raw" cheesecake, leave nuts unroasted.)
2. Line bottom and sides of square pan with 2 strips of parchment paper crosswise so they overhang rim—this will help you remove it from the pan later. (If using springform pan, no need to line it.)
3. Place nuts into food processor and blend until fine.
4. Add cranberries and grind until well mixed and is a fine texture.
5. Add 1 T. hot water and process until mixture is thick and sticky. (Add more water if necessary.)
6. Push the crust into the pan until evenly distributed at bottom. Refrigerate until filling is ready.

FILLING INSTRUCTIONS
1. Rinse and drain cashews. Place cashews, coconut oil, lemon juice, honey and vanilla extract in high-speed blender and blend until smooth and creamy.
2. Add strawberries to blender and blend again until thoroughly mixed.
3. Pour mixture onto the crust. Then push the frozen raspberries and blueberries into the filling, one at a time, dispersing throughout the filling.
4. Place cheesecake in the freezer for 4 hours or overnight. *(See serving instructions.)*

TIPS
• *Check honey resource on p. 12 for delicious, mild-tasting, creamy raw honey. It's 100% pure Canadian, well-priced, and they deliver.*

Blueberry "INSTANT" ICE CREAM

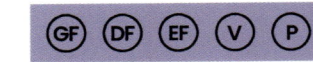

I LOVE this delicious, smooth, and fresh-tasting ice cream that is instantly made in the blender. Just throw in the frozen fruit (strawberries also amazing) with a can of coconut milk and voila!...you have soft ice cream in a couple of minutes! Using full-fat coconut milk results in a creamier ice cream texture. Add sweetener if you choose, but it's not necessary. Be creative with what you add to it or top it with. (See below for additions and topping ideas.) Or just enjoy the simple fruit flavour of the 2 ingredients. You'll be pleasantly surprised.

Makes about 6 one-cup servings

INGREDIENTS

4½ cups of **frozen blueberries** *(alternate fruit options below)*
14-oz. can **full-fat coconut milk**
Optional: 2-4 T. pure maple syrup, honey or coconut nectar

INSTRUCTIONS

1. Throw all ingredients into a good high-speed blender (such as a Blendtec or Vitamix) and blend until smooth and delicious! Serve immediately. (Can use food processor if you don't have a high-speed blender.)
2. Freeze remaining. Thaw slightly before serving.

WAYS YOU CAN ADAPT OR ENHANCE THIS RECIPE

- *Use any frozen berries (blackberries, raspberries, strawberries) ...or other frozen fruit such as mangos, peaches or cherries.*
- *Consider adding: ½ tsp. lemon zest, ¼ tsp. cardamom or ginger, or 1 T. lemon or orange liqueur.*
- *At the end of the processing, once the ice cream is smooth, try stirring in chocolate chips or cacao nibs, coconut, dried fruit, nuts (roasted hazelnuts or pecans are good), candied ginger, or lavender buds & lemon zest.*
- *Top ice cream with any fresh fruit, Lemon Curd (p.145), No-Cook Fruit Jam (p.146), coconut whipped cream, or one of the Chocolate Sauces (p.135) or Caramel Sauces (p.131-133).*
- *Easily turn this in to a smoothie or milkshake by adding more liquid (such as coconut milk, almond milk or water), to your desired consistency.*

Baked Coconut EGGNOG CUSTARD

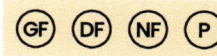

I love the flavour of custard, especially baked custard. This dairy-free coconut milk version is amazing! The nutmeg, cloves, cinnamon and vanilla are what makes it taste like eggnog. This is old world meets new age—a healthy version that is quick and easy to make. And of course, a great dessert to serve at Christmas time. At other times of the year, you may want to forego the eggnog flavour and go with vanilla. See adaptations below for Baked Coconut-Vanilla Custard version for a year-round treat.

Serves 8: Uses 1½-quart soufflé or casserole dish, or 8 individual (3") ramekins

INGREDIENTS

1-2 T. **virgin coconut oil** for greasing custard dish
5 large **eggs**
2½ cups *(1½ 14-oz. cans)* **full-fat coconut milk**
¼ cup **pure maple syrup** or honey
1 T. **pure vanilla extract**
¼ tsp. **nutmeg** *(preferably freshly grated) (and more for "dusting" top)*
pinch of **cinnamon and cloves**
Optional: ½ cup unsweetened shredded coconut

INSTRUCTIONS

1. Preheat oven to 325° F.
2. Put a kettle of water on to boil—it will be used later in recipe to create a water bath for baking.
3. Lightly grease a 1½ quart soufflé or casserole dish with coconut oil or butter. (Note: If you prefer, use individual ramekins.)
4. In an 8-cup measuring cup (or large bowl), whisk eggs for 1-2 minutes. Add coconut milk and mix well.
5. Add maple syrup, vanilla, nutmeg, cloves and cinnamon and whisk to combine.
6. If using, add grated coconut and stir well. (Coconut will rise to the top.)
7. Pour mixture into greased soufflé dish (or ramekins) and set into baking pan (such as 9x13" pan) in oven. Sprinkle extra grated nutmeg over top of custard mixture.
8. Carefully pour boiled water into the baking pan (not the custard dish) until water comes up halfway up the side of the custard dish.
9. Bake the custard for 35-40 minutes, or until set in the center (sharp knife inserted into custard center will be clean when removed). Remove from oven and cool. (Baking time will be approx. 5-10 minutes less if using individual ramekins.)
10. Serve slightly warm, room temperature, or chilled. Store covered in fridge. Keeps for several days.

WAYS YOU CAN ADAPT OR ENHANCE THIS RECIPE
• *Just before serving, drizzle a teaspoon of rum over each serving. Or heat and drizzle on warm Spiced Caramel Sauce (p.132) or Boozy Caramel Sauce (using rum) (p.133).*
• *For Baked Coconut-Vanilla Custard, omit nutmeg & cloves and instead add the scraped seeds from one vanilla bean, 1 tsp. vanilla powder, or 2 T. vanilla extract.*

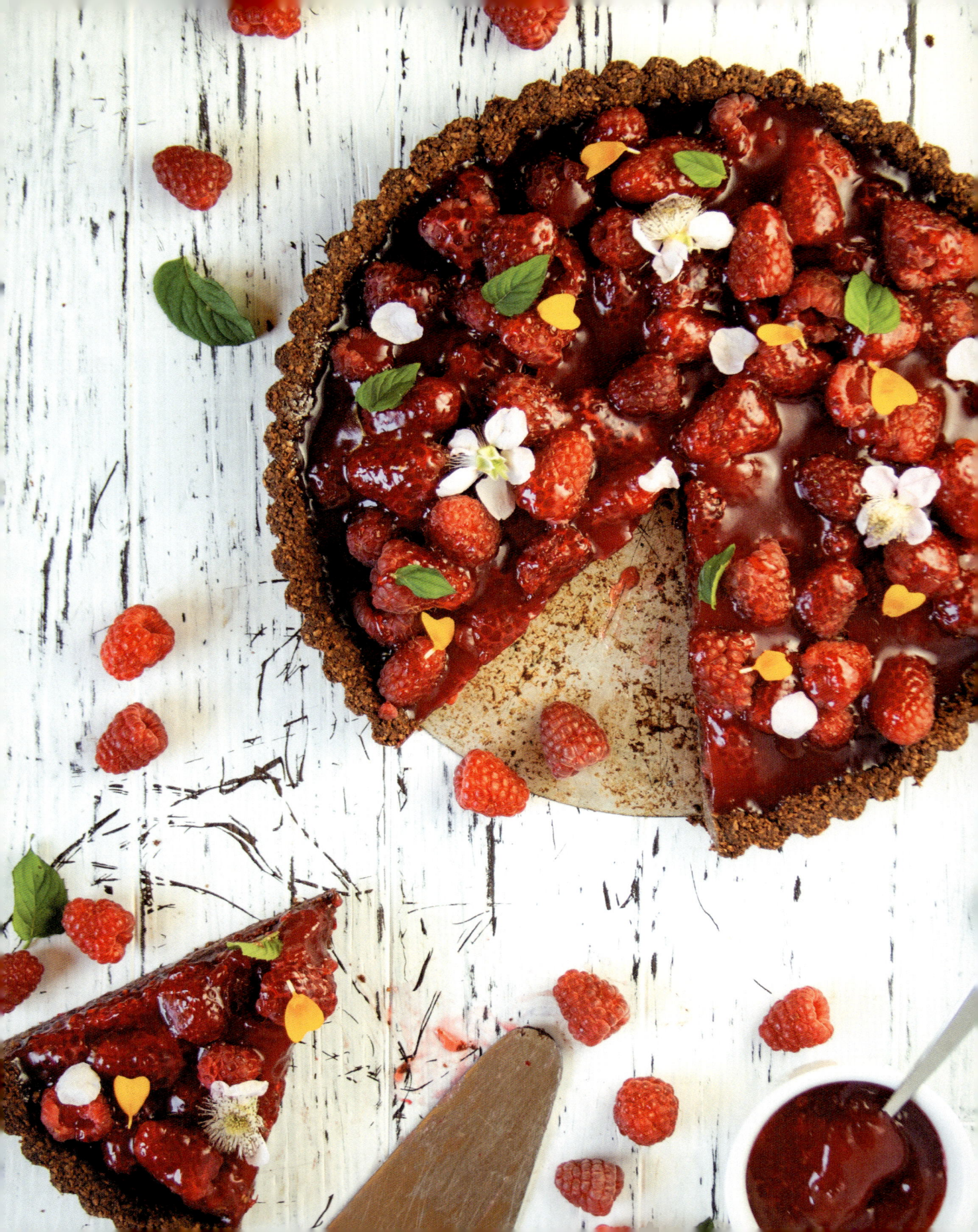

FRESH RASPBERRY PIE
with Raspberry-Honey Glaze

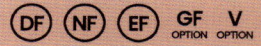

This is an old family favourite from the 1970's. We would make it every July during fresh raspberry season. It is a must-make dessert during raspberry season!! Everyone who has tried it loves it… and then they ask for the recipe. I have adapted it to make it healthier, of course. It is likely my favourite pie recipe of all time. It's so FRESH tasting because the berries are not baked…it is a no-bake pie…you just bake your favourite pie crust (or if in a rush, buy one), then fill the baked pie shell with fresh raspberries, and then pour your homemade glaze over top. Sometimes I like to add a few fresh blueberries to the pie to make it colourful and pretty. My favourite pie crust for this pie is the Easy Oil Crust (p.137); but the Butter-Vinegar Shortbread Crust (p.140) and Spelt & Butter Shortbread Crust (p.138) are also good— but use whatever crust you want. Consider making several of these fresh pies. They keep well in the fridge for 3 days. And if you can believe it, they actually freeze well. (Be sure to wrap and seal well.) Just thaw them in the fridge overnight and they are ready to serve the next day.

Makes one 9" pie *(or removable bottom tart)*, **or several tartlets**

INGREDIENTS

8" **baked pastry shell**: Easy Oil Crust (p.137), Spelt & Butter Shortbread Crust (p.138), or crust of choice
4 generous cups **fresh raspberries**, divided
¾ cup **water**
¾ tsp. **unflavoured gelatin** *(see below for V option)*
¾ cup **mild-tasting honey** *(for V: use coconut nectar)*
3 T. + 1 tsp. **organic cornstarch**
⅛ tsp. **fine sea salt**
2 tsp. **fresh lemon juice**
Optional addition: ¼ cup fresh blueberries

INSTRUCTIONS

1. Sort and arrange 3 cups (or more) of the choicest berries in a baked and cooled pastry shell. *(Optional: Add ¼ cup blueberries on top.)*
2. Crush remaining 1 cup raspberries in medium saucepan, add ¾ cup of water and simmer 3-5 minutes.
3. Strain to remove seeds and if necessary, add water to make 1 cup juice. Return juice to saucepan.
4. Measure 4 tsp. water into small bowl. Sprinkle gelatin powder on top. Let sit 10 minutes to bloom.
5. Combine cornstarch, honey and salt in separate bowl. Add to raspberry juice in saucepan. Then add dissolved gelatin. Stirring constantly, bring mixture to boil over medium heat. Turn down heat and still stirring constantly, cook until thickened and clear about 3-5 minutes.
6. Remove from heat and cool slightly (about 10 minutes). Add lemon juice and stir. (If there are any lumps, you can press the mixture through a sieve at this point.)
7. When glaze is close to room temperature (about 20-30 minutes), pour glaze over berries, coating all berries. Chill until firm. If freezing, wrap and seal pie well. Thaw in fridge overnight before serving.

WAYS YOU CAN ADAPT OR ENHANCE THIS RECIPE

- You can substitute 2 T. arrowroot flour (also called starch or powder) for the 3 T. of corn starch; but note that the texture will vary.
- Vegan option: Use coconut nectar in place of honey, and either omit the gelatin (then add 1 more T. cornstarch) or replace it with agaragar flakes (following package instructions).
- This can also be made with fresh blackberries or blueberries in place of raspberries.
- Use ⅔ cup honey if you like your glaze less sweet. Check honey resource on p.12 for delicious, mild-tasting, creamy raw honey. It's 100% pure Canadian, well-priced, and they deliver.

PARFAIT *Indulgence*

GF OPTION | **DF** OPTION | **NF** OPTION | **EF** OPTION | **V** OPTION | **P** OPTION

You've got to love a parfait. Traditionally it is laden with sugar and whipped cream. Here I offer a few healthy dairy-free and sugar-free alternatives. Basically, you can layer anything you want in a parfait glass, tall glass, or clear mug so it looks pretty. I see parfaits as layering 4 things: soft things (like puddings), fresh fruit, crunchy things like granola, nuts or seeds, and then toppings. I'm offering suggestions from recipes already in this cookbook, so you can really be creative with whatever combinations you like to make your parfaits! And to think "indulgence", in this case, means healthy! My favourite parfait combination is fresh raspberries, Vanilla & Lemon Custard Fruit Dip, broken pieces of the cookie-like baked crust from Caramel Pecan Banana Tarts, and topped with Candied Maple Walnuts (all recipes in this cookbook). But there are so many great options to choose from. Play and have fun with this!

LAYER ASSEMBLY ORDER

Layer each in serving glass carefully with a spoon so outside of glass nicely displays layers. Place in this order:

1. Fruit
2. Soft
3. Fruit
4. Crunchy
5. Coconut Whipped Cream or Strawberry Cashew Cream (p.148) *(optional)*
6. Soft
7. Crunchy
8. Topping *(optional)*

FRUIT LAYER Choose one or two:
• Fresh berries, chopped bananas, mangos, peaches, pineapple, kiwifruit, apples, pears, etc.

SOFT LAYER Choose one:
• Vanilla & Lemon Custard Fruit Dip (p.113)
• OMG! Chocolate Avocado Pudding (p.85) *(in any of the flavour options)*
• Coconut Chia Pudding (p.61)
• Lemon Curd made with Honey (p.145)
• Blueberry Sauce (p.142)
• Raspberry Coulis (p.142)
• Plain Greek Yogurt

CRUNCHY LAYER Choose one or two:
• Easy Nutty Granola (p.95)
• Crumbled baked goods such as White Chocolate Macadamia Tahini Cookies (p.37), Grandad's Oatmeal Cookies (p.35), Maple Shortbread (p.27), Almond Shortbread Fingers (p.33), Almond Oatmeal Cookies (p.36), Pecan Rice Crispy Triangles (p.39), or even baked Spelt & Butter Shortbread Crust (p.138). Or my favourite—the cookie-like baked crust from Caramel Pecan Banana Tarts (p.65).
• Nuts or seeds *(raw or roasted)*
• Buckwheat Crunchies *(see notes on p.91)*

TOPPINGS Optional. Choose one or two:
• Coconut whipped cream or Sweetened Thick Cashew Cream (p.148)
• Candied Maple Walnuts (p.108)
• One of the Chocolate Sauces (p.134-136) or Caramel Sauces (p.131-133)
• Honey-Butter Coconut Chips (p.105)
• One Apple Chip (p.110) or a Pecan Rice Crispy Triangles (p.39), placing them to stand vertically on top
• Fresh mint, lavender, or edible flowers
• More fruit

WAYS YOU CAN ADAPT OR ENHANCE THIS RECIPE
• *One of the crunchy layers can be substituted with a cake layer. Use any of the cakes in the Cakes & Cupcakes section (p.40-45).*

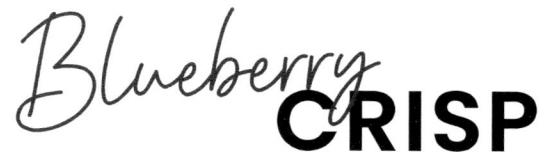
Blueberry CRISP
WITH CHOICE OF CRUMBLE TOPPING

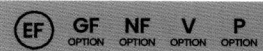

Blueberries are a Canadian staple, and as we all know, they are very healthy...they are full of nutrients and antioxidants. They are considered a Superfood, so eat up, this is another guilt-free dessert! We like this dessert especially on a cold winter night...it warms the soul. It's especially delicious served hot topped with coconut milk ice cream. I offer two toppings—one is gluten-free and grain-free (Paleo) and the other is oatmeal (with the option of making it dairy-free or vegan).

Makes 8x8" pan

BLUEBERRY BASE
6 -7 cups **fresh or frozen blueberries** (or 4 cups blueberries and 2 cups blackberries)
2 T. **tapioca** (see Tips)
zest of 1 **lemon** (optional)

CRUMBLE TOPPING OPTION 1
PALEO/GRAIN-FREE
⅓ cup **grass-fed butter**, melted
(DF & V: use coconut oil or vegan butter)
⅔ cup **almond flour**
1 cup **raw pecans**, chopped
¼ cup **coconut sugar** (or more, to taste)
1 tsp. **cinnamon**
pinch **sea salt**

CRUMBLE TOPPING OPTION 2
1 cup **rolled oats** (for GF: use GF rolled oats)
¾ cup **light spelt flour**, or flour of choice (for GF: use GF all-purpose flour mix)
½ cup **grass-fed butter**, melted (DF or V: use coconut oil or vegan butter)
⅓ cup **coconut sugar** (or more, to taste)
½ tsp. **cinnamon**
½ tsp. **cardamom**
pinch **salt**

INSTRUCTIONS
1. **Blueberry Base:** Place blueberries in an 8x8" baking pan. Sprinkle tapioca evenly over berries and then toss gently to disperse the tapioca evenly. (Or sometimes a few shakes of the pan will work.)
2. **Crumble Topping:** Mix all ingredients together in a bowl with a fork.
3. Spread the crumble topping on the blueberries and bake at 350° for 45-60 minutes, or until blueberries are cooked through and starting to bubble around edges. (If berries are frozen, you may have to bake a little longer.)
4. Remove from oven and let rest for 10 minutes. Serve with coconut ice cream or Sweetened Thick Cashew Cream (p.148).

TIPS
• Note: Tapioca is gluten-free and grain-free. This thickens the blueberry juices as it is baking. (I use Minit quick-cooking Tapioca).
• Optional: You can use a loose foil "tent" for half of the baking time to prevent topping from burning.

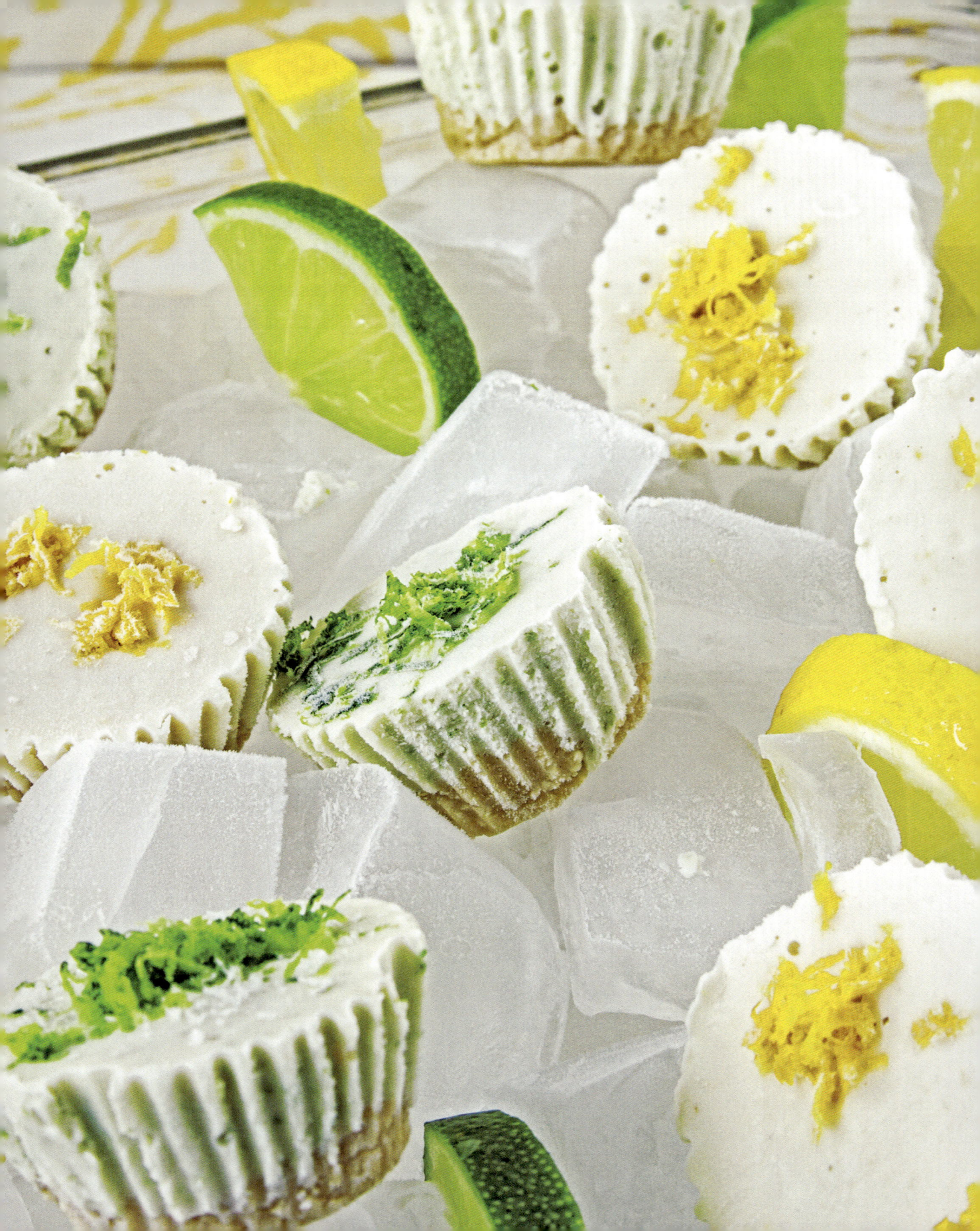

Lemon & Lime
FROZEN MINI CASHEW CHEESECAKES

These are nice little frozen bites bursting with citrus flavour. They are just perfect after a big meal. They are sweet, tart, tangy and creamy. They are easy to make and a good dessert to have on hand in the freezer for people dropping by. Thanks for this recipe, Susan.

Makes 18 mini cupcakes (or 6 regular-sized cupcakes)
Freezing Time: 2-4 hours

CRUST
½ cup **raw almonds**
2 T. **virgin coconut oil**, melted

FILLING
½ cup **raw cashews**, soaked in water for at least 2 hours or overnight in fridge, then rinse and drain
⅓ cup of **full-fat coconut milk**
¼ cup **honey** *(for V: use coconut nectar or pure maple syrup)*
4 **limes or lemons**, zested then juiced *(juice should measure approximately ¼ cup + 1 T.)*

INSTRUCTIONS
1. Line a mini muffin tin with 18 mini cupcake liners.
2. **Crust:** Place almonds and coconut oil in food processor and blend until almonds are finely ground and mixture is sticky to touch. Spoon mixture evenly between the 18 cupcake liners and push down to create a bottom crust. Place muffin pan in fridge while making filling.
3. **Filling:** Rinse and drain cashews. Place filling ingredients (including zest *and* juice) into a high-speed blender and puree until mixture is smooth and creamy.
4. Pour filling into the crusts. Optional: Top with a little extra lemon or lime zest.
5. Place muffin pan in freezer for 2-4 hours, or until frozen.
6. Serve frozen. Store in sealed container in freezer.

WAYS YOU CAN ADAPT OR ENHANCE THIS RECIPE
• I have been known to make lemon or lime frozen popsicle-type treats out of this filling. I add 1/4 tsp. lemon or lime extract plus extra 1 T. of honey to the lemon one. Makes about 4 ice pops.
• For Orange "Creamsicle" Mini Cheesecakes: Follow the recipe for Orange Creamsicles (p.109); then pour mixture over prepared crusts and freeze, as per instructions above.

Pumpkin Spice CUSTARD CUPS

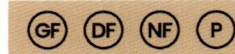

This tastes like Fall and Thanksgiving, and it's so easy to make! It's all done in the blender. Fresh pumpkin is better than canned (healthier and tastier) so if you have time, bake some ahead. Pumpkin is a kind of squash, so feel free to use leftover squash in this recipe. Butternut squash is good, but any squash will do. If using canned pumpkin, be sure to get pure pumpkin (pumpkin the only ingredient), not pumpkin pie mix. I've also included a Pumpkin Pie recipe with only two minor changes.

Makes 8 medium-sized (3") ramekins

INGREDIENTS

14-oz. can **pure, organic pumpkin puree**, or 1 ⅔ cups of cooked pumpkin or squash

14-oz. **can full-fat coconut milk**

4 **eggs**

¼ cup **pure maple syrup**, or more to taste *(or honey or coconut nectar)*

1 tsp. **pure vanilla extract** *(or ¼ tsp. vanilla bean powder)*

1 T. **pumpkin pie spice** *(see below for DIY mix)*, or more, to taste

pinch **sea salt**

PUMPKIN SPICE MIXTURE

Mix in bowl and store in sealed jar. Also use for Pumpkin Spice Latté (p.98).

- ¼ cup **cinnamon**
- 3 T. **ground ginger**
- 2 T. each of **nutmeg, cloves and allspice**

INSTRUCTIONS

1. Preheat oven to 350° F.
2. Place enough oven-safe ramekins or glass dishes to fill a 9x13" baking pan.
3. Boil water (enough for #6).
4. Place all ingredients in a blender and mix until thoroughly blended.
5. Pour the custard into ramekins.
6. Add enough boiling water to the pan to come up half way to the top of the ramekins.
7. Carefully place the pan with the ramekins and water into the oven.
8. Bake 50-60 minutes, or until a knife inserted into the center of the custard comes out clean.
9. Serve warm or chilled. This is nice served with coconut whipped cream or Thick Cashew Cream (p.148) drizzled with pure maple syrup, and then sprinkled with a few Candied Maple Walnuts (p.108) or Salty, Sweet & Spicy Maple Pecans (p.114).

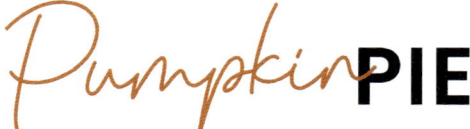

Pumpkin PIE

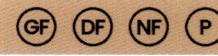

Place unbaked crust in large pie pan (I use a 9" pie pan or 11" glass tart pan) and place in fridge until filling is ready.
(Note: You can make this in to a crustless pie—see #2 below.)

INGREDIENTS
SAME AS CUSTARD CUPS, BUT WITH THESE CHANGES:

- **One Spelt & Butter Shortbread Crust** (p.138) or Crust of your choice (p.137-140)
- Decrease the **coconut milk to ½ cup**
- Increase the **maple syrup to ½ cup**

INSTRUCTIONS

1. Pour filling into prepared pie crust. Bake 350° F. for 50-60 minutes (no water bath) or until filling is set. (The time will depend on the size of your pie pan.)
2. If making a crustless pie, pour filling in to pie pan, bake and then cool to room temperature.
Then place in fridge for about 6 hours to "set" before cutting.

Pear CRUMBLE

This is an old family recipe that to this day is a feel-good, soul-food type of dessert! Of course, I have adapted it to make it healthier without losing any flavour. It's a good recipe to use up those pears that are starting to turn. It's quick to make—so dessert can be baking while you're eating dinner. Freezes well to bake later (see Tips).

Makes 8x8" pan, 4-6 servings (Can double recipe for 9x13" pan)

PEAR MIXTURE

6-6½ cups **pears**, cored & sliced—peeling is optional *(Bartlett and Anjou work well)*
2-3 T. **flour of choice** *(I use spelt flour or organic, GF all-purpose flour)*
3 T. **coconut sugar**
2 tsp. **fresh lemon juice**

TOPPING

⅓ cup **grass-fed butter**, melted *(for DF: use coconut oil.) (Or do mixture of both.)*
½ cup **flour of choice** *(I use part half GF all-purpose and half tapioca flour)*
½ cup **coconut sugar** *(add 2 T. more if you like a sweeter topping)*
⅔ cup **quick oats** *(or rolled oats)*
1½ tsp. **cinnamon**
Optional: ½ tsp. each of nutmeg, ginger and mace

INSTRUCTIONS

1. Place sliced pears into and 8x8" pan. Toss with flour, coconut sugar and lemon juice until well mixed in.
2. In a medium-sized bowl, mix topping ingredients together with a fork until well combined. Spoon topping onto pears and spread out evenly.
3. Bake 350° F. for 40-45 minutes or until pears are tender and topping is golden.
4. Serve warm or at room temperature. Nice served with coconut ice cream.

TIPS

- This freezes well before baking. After step #2, wrap pan tightly with plastic wrap then tin foil. Best to thaw in fridge 8 hours or overnight before baking.
- Use loose foil "tent" during baking if topping is getting too brown.

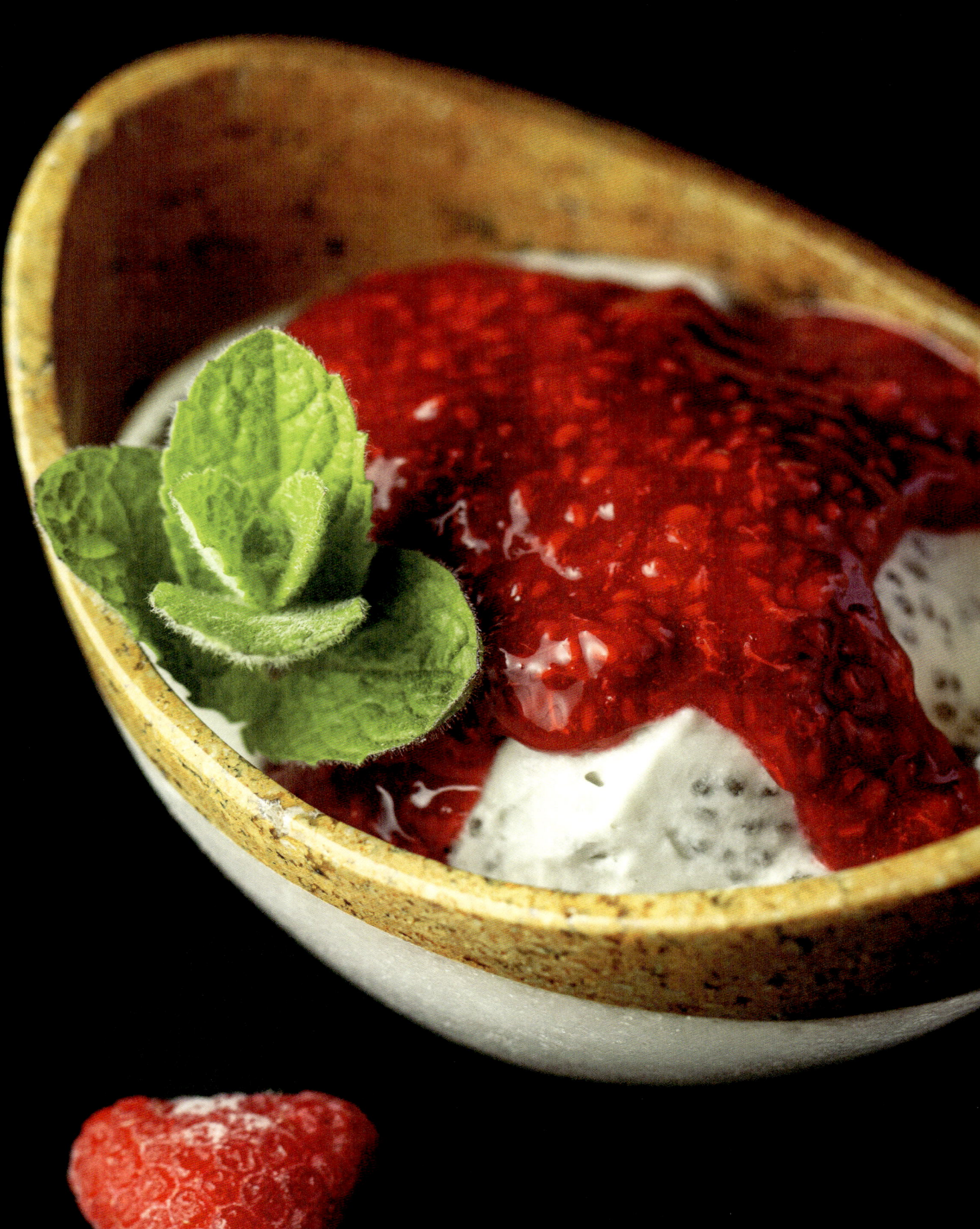

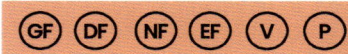

COCONUT CHIA PUDDING
with Berry Sauce

Don't let this quick and easy dessert fool you—it's delicious! (Thank you, Susan.) This 5-ingredient dessert is a great make-ahead dessert. It's delicious with raspberries or blueberries, but any berry would do.

Serves 4

INGREDIENTS
14-oz. can of **full-fat coconut milk**
2 T. **chia seeds**
4 T. **pure maple syrup** *(divided into 2)*
1 cup **fresh or frozen raspberries** or blueberries
2 tsp. **pure vanilla extract**, or less, to taste

INSTRUCTIONS
1. **Pudding:** Place coconut milk, chia seeds, and just 2 T. of the maple syrup into a blender and blend until smooth, about 5-10 seconds. Put in the fridge for 2 hours or overnight.
2. **Sauce:** Place berries, vanilla, and the other 2 T. of maple syrup into food processor and blend until mixed—chunky, not smooth.
3. **Assembly:** When ready to serve, divide the coconut mixture into 4 dessert bowls and spoon the berry sauce on top.

WAYS YOU CAN ADAPT OR ENHANCE THIS RECIPE
• Use almost any frozen fruit to create the sauce. Strawberries, blackberries, cherries, mangos, kiwi, peaches, nectarines, pineapple.
• You could also substitute berries with other fruit such as mangos, pineapple, peaches, nectarines, or kiwi fruit. If you want to make it fancier, place the dessert in clear serving glasses or martini glasses, top with coconut whipped cream, fresh berries and garnish with either toasted coconut or a sprig of mint.

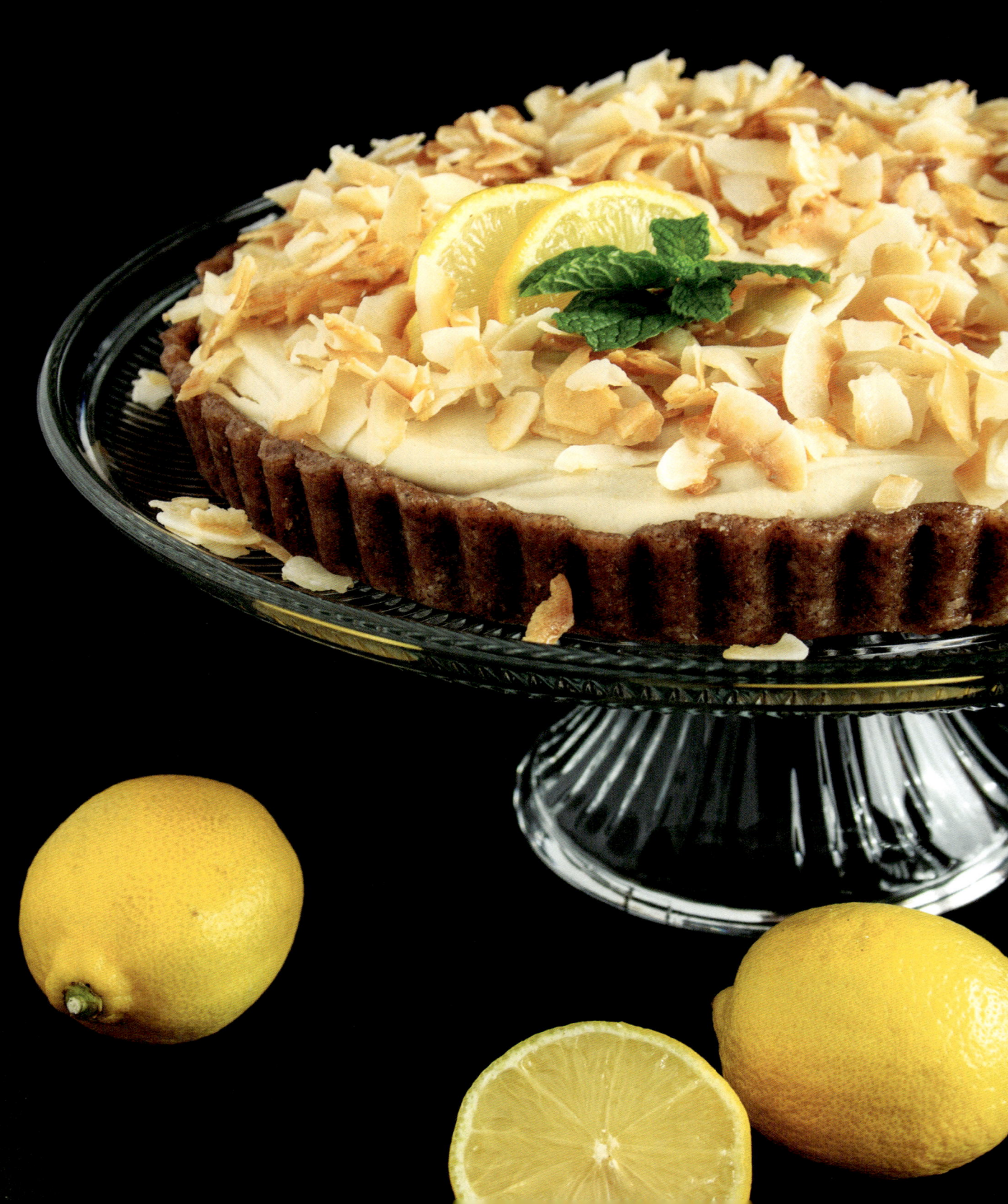

Lemon CASHEW CHEESECAKE

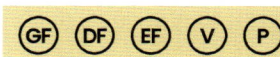

This is an impressive dessert...both in flavour and appearance. I fool people all the time—they never know this is not a cream cheese cheesecake. It's rich and creamy and very satisfying. This no-bake cheesecake is a must-do recipe in this cookbook! You'll likely make this one repeatedly, trying new toppings each time. (Topping suggestions below.) *Photo shows topping with Honey Butter Coconut Chips (p.105).*

Serves: 8-10
9" removable bottom tart pan (or 8" spring form pan)
Freezing time: Minimum 4 hours

CRUST

1½ cups **raw almonds**
⅓ cup **unsweetened shredded coconut**
2 T. **pure maple syrup** *(or honey or coconut nectar)*

FILLING

3 cups **raw cashews**, soaked in water for at least 2 hours or overnight in fridge, then rinse and drain
zest from 2 **lemons** *(approximately 1 T. packed)*
¾ cup **freshly squeezed lemon juice** *(approx. 4-5 juicy lemons)*
⅓ cup **virgin coconut oil** *(not melted)*
¾ cup **pure maple syrup**
1 tsp. **pure vanilla extract**

INSTRUCTIONS

1. **Crust:** Add almonds and coconut to food processor and run until mixture sticks together and creates a ball. Add maple syrup and blend briefly, just enough to mix it.
2. Transfer mixture to the tart pan and push crust into bottom and up sides of pan firmly. (Optional: save a few crumbs for top.) Place in the fridge while you make the filling.
3. **Filling:** Zest lemons first and then make juice. Place all filling ingredients in a highspeed blender for 60 seconds (or until it is super creamy).
4. Pour into the prepared crust and distribute evenly. Freeze. (See Tips below for freezing and serving.)
Optional: After a few hours of freezing, evenly spread Raspberry Coulis or Lemon Curd on top of frozen cheesecake and re-freeze. Top with reserved crumbs.

TIPS

• The texture is best if you put this in the freezer for a minimum of 4 hours, or overnight. If you are going to eat it after 4 hours of being in the freezer, then just remove, cut and serve, then store the remainder in the fridge. If you can, make it the day before and leave it overnight in the freezer, then remove it in the morning and place it in the fridge all day until serving in the afternoon/evening.

WAYS YOU CAN ADAPT OR ENHANCE THIS RECIPE

• *Optional: Add ⅛ tsp. of turmeric to filling for more yellow colour.*
• *You can substitute lemon with lime for a delicious Lime Cashew Cheesecake.*
• **Optional toppings:** *(Spread on top before freezing; or add to each serving when plating.)*
  • *Raspberry Coulis (p.142).*
  • *Honey Butter Coconut Chips (p.105).*
  • *Blueberry (or Strawberry or Blackberry) Sauce (p.142).*
  • *Lemon Curd made with Honey (p.145).*
  • *Some reserved crust crumbled on top.*
  • *Coconut whipped cream, lemon slices, and mint leaves (add only when serving).*

Maple Syrup PIE

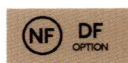

This pie is a French-Canadian tradition in maple syrup season. C'est très bon! I've created a healthy adaptation of it, and my husband, who is French-Canadian, likes it better! Don Neal is especially a fan of this pie. It is not customary to add pecans or walnuts, but if you like the idea of a "pecan maple pie", then please do—either version is absolutely delicious. Be sure try to find a quality butter, such as grass-fed or organic.

Makes one 9" pie, or a 9-10" removable bottom tart (or a few small tarts)

CRUST
Butter-Vinegar Shortbread Pie Crust (p.140),
or Spelt & Butter Shortbread Crust (p.138),
or Easy Oil Pie Crust (p.137), or other Crust of choice

FILLING
3 T. **grass-fed butter**, room temperature
(for DF: use coconut oil or vegan butter)
¾ cup **maple sugar** *(or coconut sugar)*
¾ cup **pure maple syrup**
2 **eggs**, room temperature
½ - ⅔ cup **coconut cream** *(see Tips)*, or whipping cream *(not whipped)*
1–2 T. **tapioca flour** *(also called tapioca starch)*
Optional: 1 cup raw pecan or walnut halves
(omit for NF)

CRUST INSTRUCTIONS
1. Prepare crust as per instructions and spread over bottom and sides of pie or removable bottom tart pan. Poke several holes in crust with a fork.
2. Parbake (partially bake) in preheated 400° F oven for 20 minutes. Place loose foil tent over crust to prevent edges from burning, if you like.
3. Prepare filling while crust is baking.

FILLING INSTRUCTIONS
1. Beat filling ingredients until smooth.
2. Pour mixture into the par-baked pie crust.
(If adding pecans or walnuts, sprinkle on top at this point.)
3. Place pie on cookie sheet (in case it overflows a little) and bake at 375° F for 5 minutes; then turn oven down to 325° F. and bake another 15-20 minutes. Turn oven off, leaving door closed, and let finish baking another 5-10 minutes, or until center is mostly set. (Note: filling will set more once cooled. Total baking time is 30-35 minutes.
Don't over-bake. Reduce cooking time for small tarts.)
4. Remove from oven and cool on rack. Refrigerate once pie is completely cooled.
5. Serve chilled or at room temperature.
(Optional: Serve with coconut-milk whipped cream.)

TIPS
• Coconut cream is the solid part of a can of full-fat coconut milk. It's easiest to separate the coconut cream from the coconut milk if the can is refrigerated overnight. (Always keep a can in the fridge!)

Caramel Pecan BANANA TARTS

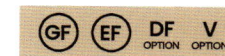

Warning: Addictive! Imagine this—a crunchy cookie-like crust topped with fresh bananas, roasted pecans and topped with caramel sauce. Decadent! I had fun creating these. Perhaps too much fun! If you like a chocolate-pecan-caramel combination, check out the "Turtle" Tarts option below—a sweet and decadent treat.

Makes 9-12 tarts (muffin size) (Or makes 24-30 mini tarts using mini muffin pan)

CRUST
- 1 cup plus 2 T. **almond meal or almond flour**
- ½ cup **raw pecans**
- 2 tsp. **coconut flour**
- 2 T. **coconut sugar**
- 2½ T. **grass-fed butter**, melted *(for DF & V: use coconut oil or vegan butter)*
- 1 tsp. **cinnamon**
- pinch **sea salt** *(optional)*

FILLING
- 2-3 ripe, firm **bananas** *(Do not cut banana until all ingredients are cooled and ready to assemble so bananas don't oxidize and turn brown.)*
- 1¼ cups **raw pecans**, chopped

TOPPING
Almond Butter Caramel Sauce (p.131) *(or your choice of caramel sauce to equal about 1 cup)*

INSTRUCTIONS
1. Preheat oven to 375° F. Line muffin pan with 9-12 silicone or paper muffin liners.
2. **Crust:** Place all crust ingredients in a food processor fit with an S-blade and process for about 15-20 seconds or until mixture resembles a mealy texture (until butter is mixed in and there are no large chunks of nuts).
3. Divide crust evenly into muffin cups and press down firmly to create a solid base. Bake for 7 minutes or until golden brown. Let cool completely while making the filling and topping. *Note: Keep cooked crust in muffin pans for assembly and chilling.*
4. **Topping: a)** While oven is still on, roast chopped pecans for 4-6 minutes. (Watch carefully—they burn quickly!) **b)** Prepare the caramel sauce as per the recipe. Remove caramel sauce from heat to let cool for about 15-20 minutes, or until sauce becomes thicker.
5. **Filling:** When ready to assemble the tarts, slice the banana into one-inch pieces; then cut each piece into small chunks, the size of green peas.
6. **Assembly:** Place banana chunks into one cooled tart crust. Do this into the rest of the tarts. Sprinkle each tart with the roasted pecans. Then pour or spoon the caramel sauce over top each tart.
7. Refrigerate 2 hours or until completely set. Serve cold or at room temperature. Tarts can be left at room temperature for up to 2 hours. Store in fridge for 2-3 days.

WAYS YOU CAN ADAPT OR ENHANCE THIS RECIPE
- *For Turtle Tarts, simply swap the bananas for a double batch of Chocolate Chili Ganache (p.136), omitting the spices. Place chocolate ganache into bottom of baked and cooled tart shell. Let set in fridge for 10-15 minutes. Then top with roasted pecans and caramel sauce.*
- *Boozy Version: Whisk in 1-2 T. Whiskey, Bourbon or Amaretto into the Caramel Sauce.*
- *Salted Caramel Version: After assembly (or when serving), top each tart with pinch of fleur de sel or flaked sea salt (such as Maldon).*

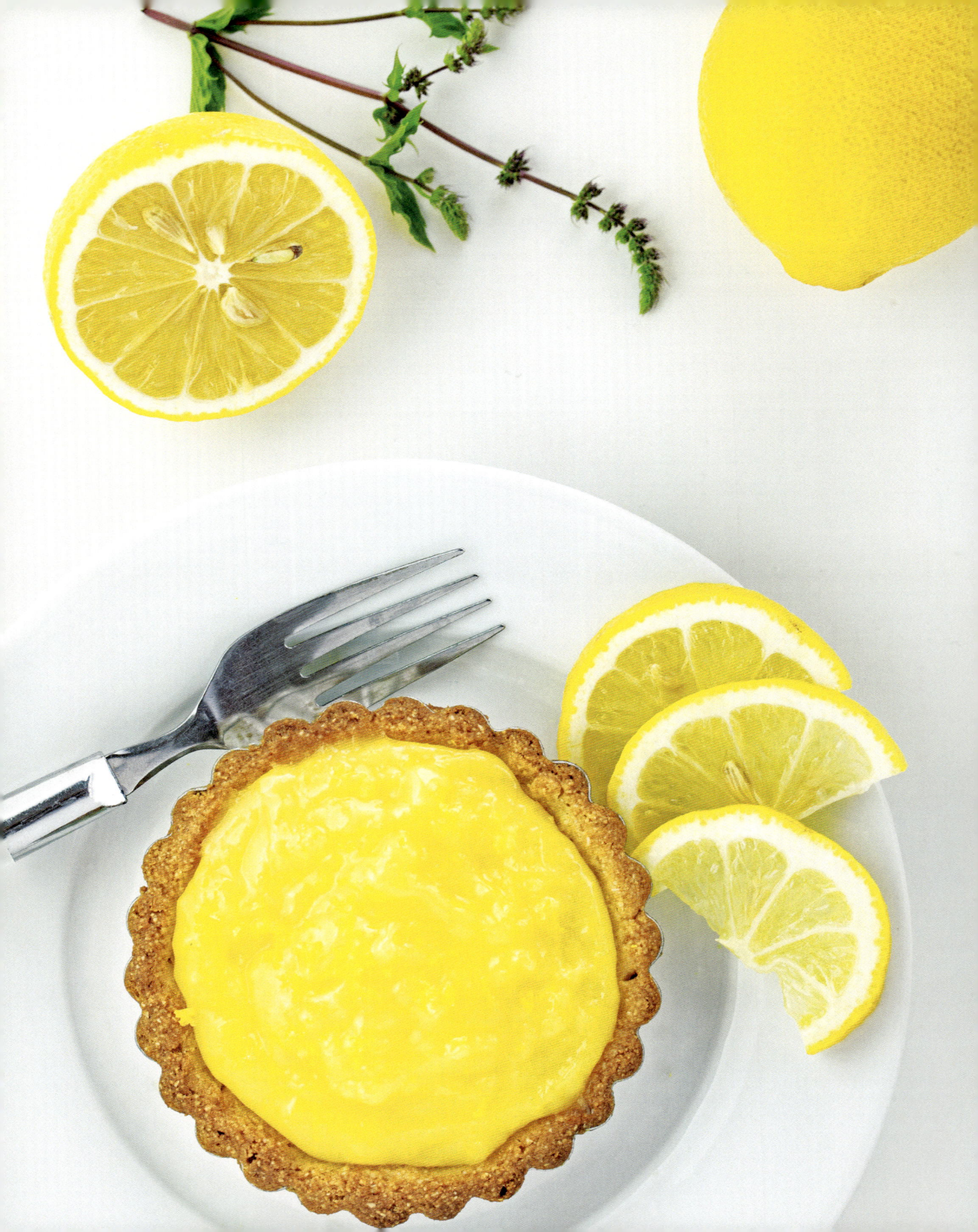

Lemon TARTS

I don't know one single person who doesn't love lemon desserts. And this one tops them all...it's so lemony, tart, and has just enough sweetener to please the palate. You could put meringue on them and make lemon meringue tarts, if you like. You can also make this into a pie, if you prefer.
Choose your favorite crust...several options are provided.

Makes 6-8 tarts, depending on size of your tart shells (or one pie)

INGREDIENTS

One "baked" pie crust of choice:
Butter-Vinegar Shortbread Crust (p.140),
or Spelt & Butter Shortbread Crust (p.138),
For GF: use Pecan Oat Crust (p.139)
For DF, use Easy Oil Crust (p.137)

One batch of Lemon Curd made with Honey (p.145)

INSTRUCTIONS

1. Make the crust of choice into tart shells and be sure it is blind baked (pre-baked) and cooled to room temperature.
2. Make the lemon curd and let cool to room temperature.
3. Spoon or pipe lemon curd into tart shells. Preferable to eat immediately. If not eating right away, cover and refrigerate.

TIPS
• *I use 3" removable bottom tart shells, but you can use what you have.*

WAYS YOU CAN ADAPT OR ENHANCE THIS RECIPE
• *These tarts lend themselves well to a grain-free, gluten-free, dairy-free and Paleo crust using a simple cassava flour crust—see Otto's Naturals website for recipe.*
• *Topping suggestions: Coconut Whipped Cream, Thick Cashew Cream or Strawberry Cashew Cream (p.148), Mint sprigs, Lemon zest curLs, Fresh berries, a toasted meringue or an Italian meringue made with Honey, Dollop of Raspberry Coulis (p.142) or Blueberry Sauce (p.142).*

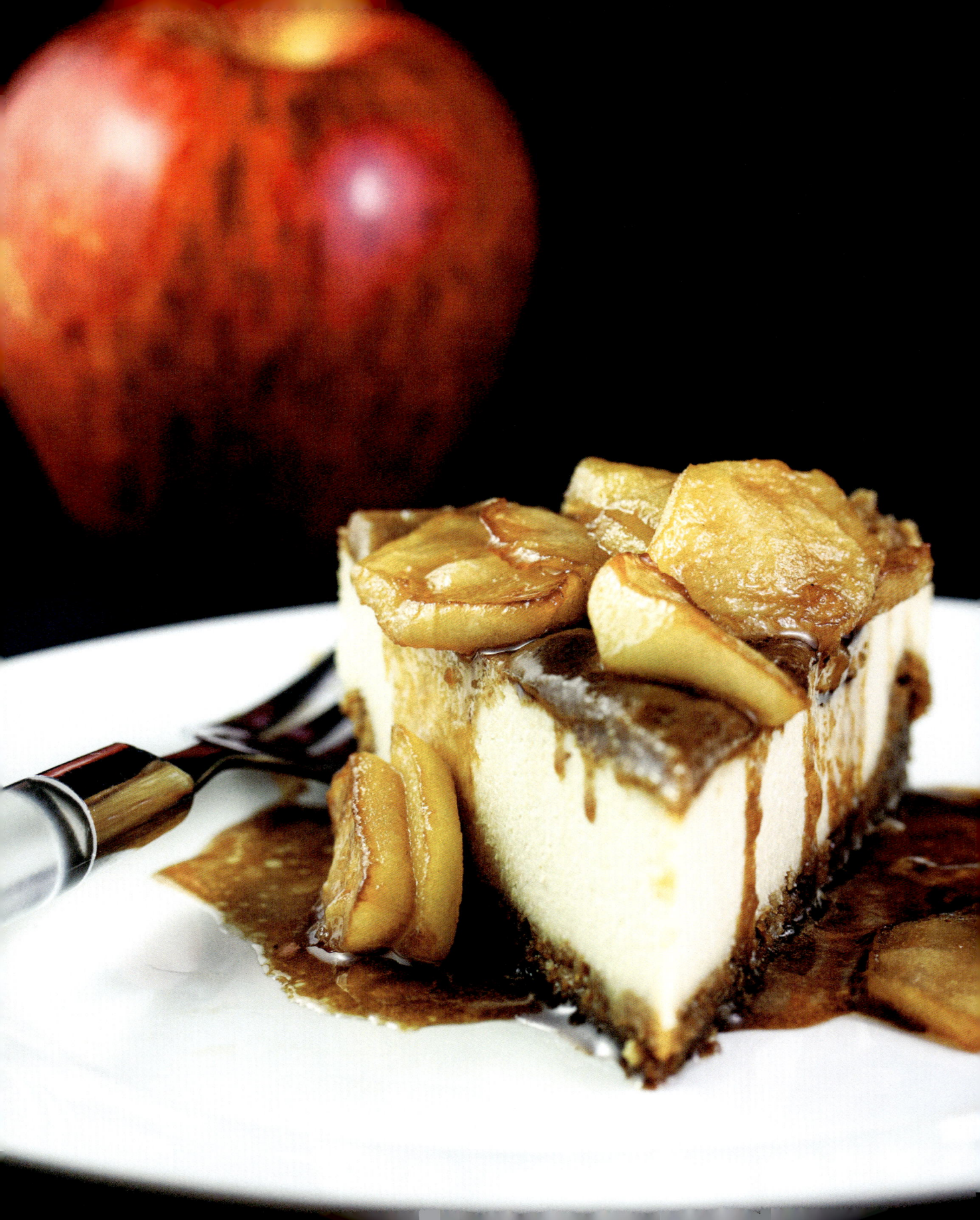

BAKED CASHEW CHEESECAKE
with Caramelized Apples

A non-dairy baked New York style cheesecake to die for. You would never know it's non-dairy—it is still rich and creamy. You would also never know it contains a vegetable! Filling ingredients are all done in a blender. This is a versatile baked cheesecake recipe that can be served with a variety of toppings—be sure to try them out (see list below).

Serves 12 (makes 9" springform pan)

INGREDIENTS

One unbaked Graham Crust (p.139)
or partially baked Spelt & Butter Shortbread Crust (p.138)
Caramelized Apples (p.141)
(Note: One batch is 4 servings, so double or triple batch as needed.)
1 cup **raw cashews**, soaked in water for at least 2 hours or overnight in fridge, then rinse and drain
8 oz *(225g)* **zucchini**, peeled and chopped
½ cup **virgin coconut oil**
2 T. **grass-fed butter** *(for DF: use vegan butter)*
½ cup + 1 T. **coconut cream**—the solid part from a can of full-fat coconut milk *(also see Tips)*
½ cup **honey** *(or more, to taste—see Adaptations below)*
¼ cup **freshly squeezed lemon juice**
3 **eggs**
1½ tsp. **pure vanilla extract**
3 T. **arrowroot flour** *(also called arrowroot starch or powder)*

ALTERNATIVE CHEESECAKE TOPPINGS

Spread topping of choice on top of cheesecake and then cut to serve. Alternatively, cut and serve with topping drizzled on top of each cheesecake slice.

- Caramel Sauce (p.131-133) or Pumpkin Spice Caramel Sauce (p.133) Serve with pinch of fleur de sel or flaked sea salt for "salted caramel".
- Blueberry Sauce (or strawberry, blackberry, berry of choice) (p.142)
- Raspberry Coulis (p.142)
- Chocolate Sauce or Ganache of choice (p.134-136)
- Lemon Curd made with Honey (p.145)
- Caramelized Bananas, Pears, Peaches or Mangos (p.141)
- Honey Butter Coconut Chips (p.105) (place on top of one of the sauces)

INSTRUCTIONS

1. Ahead of time: Soak cashews overnight.
2. Preheat oven to 350° F. Rinse and drain cashews. Boil water (for step #6).
3. Press Graham Pecan Oat Crust firmly into bottom of springform pan. Refrigerate until filling is ready.
4. Combine all filling ingredients in a high-speed blender and blend until smooth and creamy.
5. Pour filling over prepared crust. Place the springform pan on a piece of foil inside a baking pan and wrap foil up sides of springform pan tightly.
6. Put the foil-covered springform pan in a larger baking pan or dish, such as 9x13". Then fill this dish with approximately 3 cups boiling water. Be careful not to get any water in the cheesecake pan. (Baking in a water bath provides better results.)
7. Carefully place the whole baking dish in oven on middle rack. Bake 20 minutes at 350° F, then reduce heat to 250° F and bake an additional 90 minutes, until the center is completely set.
8. Turn oven off and crack the door to allow the cake to cool slowly. Leave for about 1 hour (cooling cake slowly prevents cracks in top of the cake). When the cake is cool enough to handle, remove it from the oven and let cool to room temperature.
9. Transfer cake to fridge and chill 6 hours, or overnight, to fully set.
10. To serve, top with Caramelized Apples or one of the Alternative Topping suggestions provided.
11. Wrap and refrigerate for up to 4 days.

TIPS
- Refrigerate a can of full-fat coconut milk; the coconut cream solidifies and makes it easier to remove. (Save the remaining liquid for smoothies or lattés!) Always keep a can of full-fat coconut milk in the fridge.

WAYS YOU CAN ADAPT OR ENHANCE THIS RECIPE:
- This is not a sweet cheesecake, so feel free to increase sweetener to your liking. Or be sure to add a generous amount of one or more toppings. (Or create a buffet of various topping for your guests to serve themselves.)

CHOCOLATE

See Recipe Index for full list of recipes containing chocolate.

Brown Butter & Rosemary Chocolate Tartlets with Sea Salt *71*

Peanut Butter Chocolate Nib'd Truffles *73*

Patti's Peppermint Patties *74*

Chocolate Bark with Various Toppings *75*

Fudgy Butternut Squash Espresso Brownies *77*

Nutella Truffles & Nutella Chocolate Cups *78*

Coconut Clouds in Dark Chocolate *79*

Chocolate & Chili Quinoa Cake with Chocolate-Chili Ganache *81*

Chocolate Espresso Pâté *82*

Chocolate Espresso Ganache Tart *83*

OMG! Chocolate Avocado Puddings *85*

Flourless Chocolate Cake *86*
with Raspberry Coulis
with Whiskey Caramel Sauce
with Sugarless Chocolate Frosting

Dark Chocolate Pecan Clusters with Sea Salt *87*

Chocolate Chevre Truffles – 3 Ways *89*

Crunchy Chocolate Bites *91*
(cover photo)

Brown Butter & Rosemary
CHOCOLATE TARTLETS
WITH SEA SALT

GF | EF | V | P | DF OPTION | V OPTION

If you like chocolate, you'll love these 2-bite treats! This is my fave chocolate in the cookbook. The combination of brown butter, rosemary and chocolate is heavenly!! This is an easy and quick recipe to make. Don't be fooled by the brown butter…it only takes a few minutes to make. However, if you want you can substitute extra-virgin olive oil for the butter. They are a nice bite-size treat to enjoy with coffee, for an afternoon snack, or for a quick and healthy dessert. If you don't have fresh rosemary, just leave it out and you have a delicious Brown Butter Chocolate Tart (with optional sea salt).

Makes 24 mini tarts

CRUST

1 cup plus 2 T. **almond flour** *(or other finely ground raw nut such as pecans, walnuts or hazelnuts)*

¼ cup **unsweetened shredded coconut** *(be sure it's finely shredded—see Tips)*

3 T. good quality **cacao powder** *(preferably raw organic)*

2 T. **pure maple syrup**

¼ cup **virgin coconut oil**, melted

pinch **sea salt**

FILLING

½ cup **grass-fed butter** made in to brown butter *(see Tips) (for V & DF: use extra virgin olive oil)*

⅓ cup plus 2 T. **pure maple syrup**

1 cup good quality **cacao powder** *(preferably raw, organic)*, sifted first if there are lumps

2 T. finely minced **fresh rosemary** *(Do not use rosemary powder. Fresh rosemary is best for this recipe. Or rosemary can be omitted or substituted with fresh sage.)*

Optional Topping:

1 T. chopped, **fresh rosemary**

Pinch of **flaked sea salt** for each tart

INSTRUCTIONS

1. **Crust:** In medium bowl, combine first 3 ingredients with fork so there are no lumps.
2. Add next 3 ingredients and blend well with fork.
3. Divide dough evenly (approx. 2 tsp. in each) among 24 mini paper cupcake liners (using a mini muffin pan to hold) and press into bottom evenly and firmly. Refrigerate until filling is ready.
4. **Filling:** Add the filling ingredients to large bowl and whisk well to blend until smooth and light. (Or use hand mixer or food processor.) Taste at this point and add 1 or 2 T. more of maple syrup, if desired.
5. Pour or spoon approximately 2 tsp. of filling onto the crusts and spread evenly.
6. **Optional Topping:** Sprinkle extra chopped rosemary on top. If you happen to have rosemary flowers in season, use as a pretty garnish. And/or sprinkle with fleur de sel or flaked sea salt.
7. Refrigerate tarts to set and firm for 1-2 hours. (Note: The brown butter flavour is enhanced at room temperature. Ideally, let tartlets sit out for 30 minutes before eating.)
8. Store in airtight container in fridge for up to a week.

TIPS

- *You can always pulse coconut in blender or food processor to make it finely shredded.*
- *Brown butter is simply butter that is cooked gently in a saucepan that turns golden brown in colour. It creates an accelerated butter flavour—slightly nutty and caramelized. Simple instructions: In a medium saucepan, melt butter over medium-low heat. Cook until butter takes on a light brown color and nutty aroma—about 5-10 minutes. (Or use online video instructions.)*

WAYS YOU CAN ADAPT OR ENHANCE THIS RECIPE

- *Substitute rosemary with fresh sage*
- *For an impressive dessert for company, you can make these bigger into 6-8 regular-sized cupcake/muffin liners.*

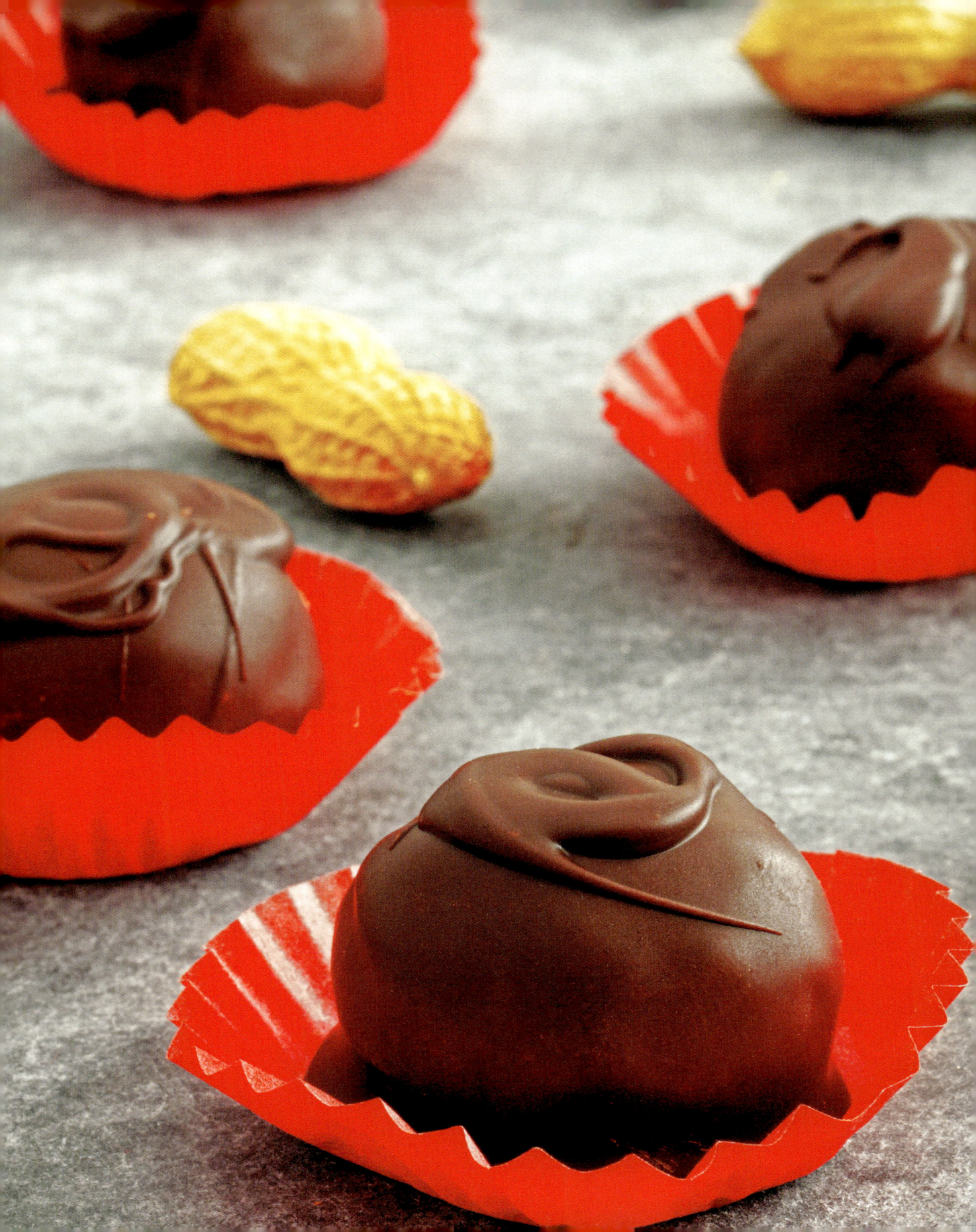

Peanut Butter CHOCOLATE NIB'D TRUFFLES

(GF) (EF) (P) DF OPTION V OPTION

These are everyone's favourites. They taste like Reese's Peanut Butter Cups...but better! They are healthier and less sweet. I have adapted this recipe from an old family recipe. We used to always make these at Christmas time, and for many years I've been giving them as gifts. Now I make them all year round! These completely satisfy the craving for that peanut butter and chocolate combination! They are crunchy and smooth, and are filled with protein, healthy fats, and one of the best antioxidants out there—raw cacao nibs. Enjoy!

Makes 36-42 truffles

TRUFFLE
1 cup **crunchy peanut butter**
¼ cup **honey** (for V: see Adaptations below)
½ cup **cacao nibs**
¼ cup **melted butter or homemade ghee** (for V & DF: see Adaptations)
2 T. **coconut flour**

COATING
1½ cups **dark/bittersweet chocolate chips** (70-85% cacao) (or 9 oz/260g dark baking chocolate, chopped) (see Adaptations below for refined sugar-free chocolate)

INSTRUCTIONS
1. Stir together peanut butter, honey, cacao nibs, melted better, and coconut flour in a medium sized bowl until well-combined.
2. Place in fridge for 30 minutes or more until firm.
3. Roll into one-inch balls and place on parchment-lined cookie sheet in fridge or freezer for another 30-60 minutes.
4. Melt chocolate chips slowly in a bain marie (in a bowl over simmering water— don't let bowl touch water).
5. Using one fork and one small spoon, dip frozen truffles in melted chocolate to cover truffles completely. Gently tap fork on side of bowl to remove excess chocolate and then place on parchment-lined cookie sheet.
6. Chill in fridge until set. Store in fridge or freezer.

WAYS YOU CAN ADAPT OR ENHANCE THIS RECIPE
• V options: Replace honey with coconut nectar; and replace butter or ghee with coconut oil or vegan butter.
• For refined sugar-free chocolate coating, use unsweetened chocolate and melt with 2 tsp. of coconut oil or homemade ghee. Remove from heat and whisk in 2 T. maple syrup or honey.
• Any extra melted chocolate you may have can be drizzled over top of the dipped truffles. Or drizzle on melted white or milk chocolate for pretty contrast.

Patti's PEPPERMINT PATTIES

GF | DF | EF | P | V OPTION

These taste like the real deal! It surprises people how good they are. And go figure that they are also good for you: healthy fats, antioxidants, fibre, vitamins and minerals. A two-stage, easy recipe. Place a few peppermint patties in a small box with coloured tissue for a great gift.

Makes about 12

PEPPERMINT FILLING

½ cup **blanched almond flour**
3 T. **arrowroot flour** *(also called starch or powder)*
2 T. **honey** *(for V: use 3 T. coconut nectar)*
2 T. **virgin coconut oil**, or homemade ghee, melted
2 T. **coconut cream** *(the solid part from a can of full-fat coconut milk)*
3 - 4 drops **food grade peppermint essential oil** *(or ¾ tsp. good quality peppermint extract)*

CHOCOLATE COATING

100 g *(3½ oz.)* **dark chocolate chunks or chips** *(preferably 70-85% cacao)*
½ tsp. **virgin coconut oil** *(or homemade ghee or vegan butter) (see Adaptations below)*

INSTRUCTIONS

1. Combine all Peppermint Filling ingredients in a bowl and stir to combine thoroughly. Taste at this point and add more peppermint, if desired.
2. Place bowl in fridge for 2-3 hours for mixture to harden slightly.
3. Roll in to small balls, then gently flatten into patties. Freeze on parchment-lined baking sheet for at least 1 hour.
4. Place Chocolate Coating ingredients in a bowl over simmering water. Then remove from heat and let stand 5-10 minutes.
5. Dip each pattie into chocolate and toss to coat. Tap excess chocolate off before transferring back to the lined baking sheet. Let set in fridge. Store in sealed container in the fridge for up to 2 weeks.

TIPS
• If you have excess chocolate after dipping all the patties, you can re-dip after chilling the peppermint patties for about 20 minutes. Or you can drizzle the excess chocolate on top of the patties.
• Use good quality mint extract such as "Simply Organic" brand.

WAYS YOU CAN ADAPT OR ENHANCE THIS RECIPE
• For refined sugar-free chocolate coating, use unsweetened chocolate and melt with 1 tsp. of coconut oil (or homemade ghee or vegan butter). Remove from heat and whisk in 2 T. maple syrup or honey.

Chocolate BARK
WITH VARIOUS TOPPINGS

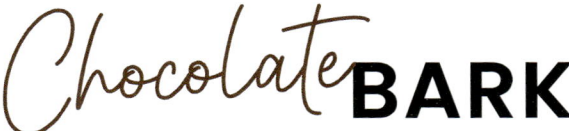

Also called French Chocolate Bark. A few topping choices are offered, but you can actually sprinkle any dried fruit or nuts on top and it would be delicious. It's always good no matter what! And it makes a great gift. Did I mention how easy this is to make? Be sure to check out the Mendiants method, below. You can temper your chocolate *(see Tips)*; it is not necessary for this recipe, but will result in a slightly better product.

INGREDIENTS
8 oz *(225g)* **good quality dark/bittersweet chocolate** *(70-85% cacao)*, chopped

TOPPING CHOICES (CHOOSE ONE)
1. CHERRY-ALMOND-COFFEE:
2 tsp. finely ground coffee *(grind beans yourself for best flavour)*, ¼ cup chopped, dried tart cherries, ⅓ cup raw almonds *(roasted and chopped in half)*, ¼ tsp. cinnamon, and 1-2 pinches of course or flaked sea salt or fleur de sel. If desired, top with a few extra roasted almonds. *(Note: can use decaffeinated coffee beans, if desired.)*

2. CHRISTMAS: ⅓ cup each of goji berries *(or dried cranberries)*, roasted hazelnuts, pumpkin seeds, slivered almonds, and 2 T. candied ginger, chopped.

3. GRANOLA: 1 cup Easy Nutty Granola (p.95).

4. FRENCH (NUTS & FRUIT): ½ cup of any of these chopped, dried fruits: apricots, cranberries, raisins, figs or candied orange peel. And ½ cup of any of these roasted nuts: cashews, almonds, pecans, macadamia nuts or pistachios. You can stir in the nuts instead of placing on top, if you wish.

INSTRUCTIONS
1. Line cookie sheet with parchment paper.
2. Slowly melt chocolate in a bain marie (in double boiler or in a bowl over simmering water—don't let bowl touch water). (Temper chocolate if you wish—see Tips.)
3. Pour melted chocolate into a large slab onto the parchment-lined cookie sheet, spreading evenly.
4. Sprinkle rest of ingredients on top.
5. Place in fridge 1-2 hours, or until set.
6. Break into pieces.
7. Keep stored in seal container in the fridge for 2-3 weeks.

TIPS
• Tempering is a method of heating then cooling chocolate so it becomes shiny and hard. Look online for instructions.

WAYS YOU CAN ADAPT OR ENHANCE THIS RECIPE
• Drop the melted chocolate into 1" circles on parchment and place nuts and dried fruit on each circle. (These are called Mendiants. Especially popular with the French.)
• Salted chocolate is delicious. Try sprinkling bark with a small amount of fleur de sel or flaked sea salt.
• For refined sugar-free version, substitute bittersweet chocolate with good quality unsweetened chocolate and melt with 1 tsp. virgin coconut oil or homemade ghee. Remove from heat and whisk in 2 T. maple syrup or honey.
• For NF: Omit nuts or substitute nuts with pumpkin seeds.

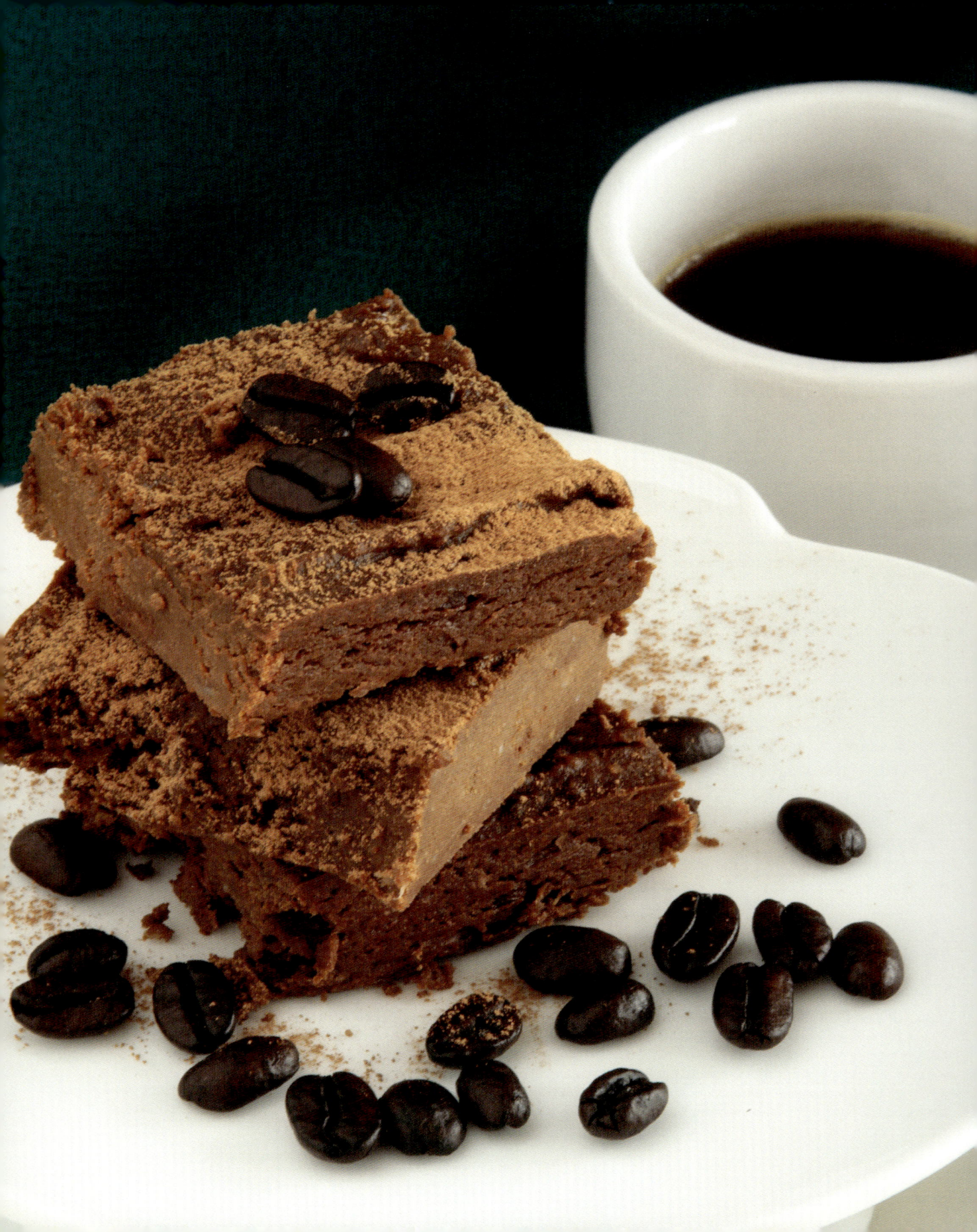

Fudgy Butternut Squash ESPRESSO BROWNIES

GF | DF | P | NF OPTION

These sugarless brownies are my favourite brownies of all time. The intense chocolate and espresso flavour makes this a hit with coffee lovers. And to think this treat has one cup of vegetables and no added sweeteners…it's only sweetened with dates. (These are not very sweet, as brownies often are, but they do, indeed, satisfy the sweet tooth.) Add almond meal (fibre, protein & vitamins) and healthy fats and you have a crazy-healthy-good dessert. The added ground espresso beans and chocolate chips make for a rich chocolate and coffee flavour. (See Adaptations below for a version without coffee.)

Makes 16 squares in 8x8" pan

INGREDIENTS

½ cup **brewed espresso** or strong coffee *(can use decaffeinated)*
1 cup **dates**, pits removed and roughly chopped
½ cup **virgin coconut oil**, melted, cooled to room temperature
1 cup **cooked butternut squash** *(see Adaptations below)*
½ cup **cacao powder** *(preferably raw, organic)*
1 T. **coconut flour**
1 **egg**, room temperature
½ cup **almond meal or almond flour** *(for NF: use ⅔ cup cooked quinoa)*
1½ tsp. **pure vanilla extract**
pinch **sea salt**
3 T. **espresso or coffee beans**, very finely ground *(better flavour if you grind beans yourself)*
½ cup **dark chocolate chips** *(or cacao nibs) (optional)*

INSTRUCTIONS

1. Cook butternut squash.
2. Bring coffee and dates to boil in small pan. Turn heat to low simmer to soften dates for 10 minutes. Let cool to room temperature. Save ¼ cup of reduced liquid and include in recipe.
3. Melt coconut oil and let cool.
4. Preheat oven to 350° F and liberally grease an 8x8" baking pan with coconut oil.
5. Put all items except chocolate chips and espresso beans in food processor, blending one item at a time before adding the next. Blend until smooth.
6. Stir in chocolate chips and espresso beans.
7. Pour into prepared pan.
8. Bake approximately 30 minutes, or until cooked through. Note: It will be soft while hot.
9. Let cool, then refrigerate. Cut and serve once it is chilled. Store in covered container in fridge for up to 1 week.

WAYS YOU CAN ADAPT OR ENHANCE THIS RECIPE

- Squash: You can substitute butternut squash with cooked carrot, sweet potato or yam.
- If you use cacao nibs (instead of chocolate chips to avoid sugar), these brownies will be less sweet. In this case, you may want to add another ¼ cup of dates. Cacao nibs or chocolate chips can also be substituted with chopped walnuts or pecans.
- For a decadent dessert: Cut an extra-large square of brownie and place on a plate. Then drizzle brownie and plate with slightly warmed Caramel Sauce (p.131-133) (for a "Salted Caramel" experience, sprinkle a pinch of flaked sea salt on top). Or try drizzle of warm Chocolate Sauce (p.134-136) or chilled Raspberry (or Mango) Coulis (p.142). Consider adding a dollop of coconut whipped cream. Sprinkle with chopped, roasted hazelnuts or cacao nibs. Add a few fresh berries to the plate.
- Coffee: Feel free to substitute with decaffeinated coffee beans. Children may not like the coffee flavour—so omit the ground coffee and instead soak/heat the dates in ½ cup water or orange juice. Add some orange zest to the batter, if desired.

"Nutella" TRUFFLES

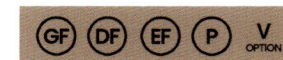

This is one of the many recipes that came out of "playing" with my homemade Nutella (Hazel-Nut-Ella Chocolate Spread). It makes a beautiful gift (wrap in small confection box) or can be served at the end of a meal. I admit, I have one or two in the morning with my cup of coffee when I most enjoy chocolate. Pure indulgence. Pure heaven! The Italians would be proud.

Makes about 12

INGREDIENTS

2 cups of **homemade Nutella**
(Hazel-Nut-Ella Chocolate Spread, p.144), chilled
1 ⅓ cups *(200g)* **dark/bittersweet chocolate chips**
(70-85% cacao) or baking chocolate *(see Adaptations)*
Optional: ½ cup **whole, raw hazelnuts** *(roasted 350° F. oven for 10 mins.)*

INSTRUCTIONS

1. Be sure your homemade Nutella is refrigerated for this first step. If necessary, place Nutella in freezer for 10 minutes. Roll Nutella mixture into 1" balls and place on a baking sheet lined with parchment or wax paper. Freeze for at least 1 hour.
2. Melt chocolate in a bain marie (in a bowl over a pot of simmering water—don't let bowl touch water).
3. Using two small spoons or forks, dip frozen truffle-balls one at a time into warm melted chocolate. Let excess chocolate drain off, then place onto parchment-lined cookie sheet.
4. Optional: At this point, you can push one whole roasted hazelnut in centre of each ball before chilling. This is similar to a traditional Gianduja—a popular Italian Hazelnut Chocolate Truffle.
5. Refrigerate until set, 30-60 minutes. Store in sealed container for up to 2 weeks.

WAYS YOU CAN ADAPT OR ENHANCE THIS RECIPE
• *For refined sugar-free chocolate, substitute with unsweetened chocolate and melt with 2 tsp. of virgin coconut oil or homemade ghee. Remove from heat and whisk in 2 T. pure maple syrup or honey.*

"Nutella" CHOCOLATE CUPS

INSTRUCTIONS

1. Make Mini Chocolate Cups according to recipe on page 120.
2. Fill with spoonful of room temperature Hazel-Nut-Ella Chocolate Spread (p.144).
3. Optional: Sprinkle each with a pinch of chopped, roasted hazelnuts or top with one whole roasted hazelnut.
4. Store in sealed container in fridge for up to 2 weeks.
4. **Optional:** At this point, you can push one whole roasted hazelnut in centre of each ball before chilling. This is similar to a traditional Gianduja—Italian Hazelnut Chocolate Truffles. Or place hazelnut on top.
5. Refrigerate until set, 30-60 minutes. Store in sealed container for up to 2 weeks.

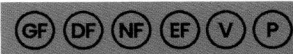

COCONUT CLOUDS
in Dark Chocolate

These truffles are like a coconut chocolate bar (think Almond Joy or Bounty), but are made with pure ingredients, of course! When you bite into them, they look like clouds and taste like heaven—hence the name. Easy enough to make with children. Another quick and easy recipe. Thanks for the inspiration, Susan.

Makes 18-24 truffles

TRUFFLE CENTERS
2½ cups **unsweetened, shredded coconut**
2 T. **virgin coconut oil** *(can use a little more, if needed)*
2 T. **honey** *(for V: use coconut nectar)*
Optional: flavour additions, see Adaptations below

CHOCOLATE COATING
(see adaptations for using melted dark chocolate)
⅔ cup (80g/2.8oz.) **cacao butter**
⅔ cup **cacao powder** *(preferably raw, organic)*
⅓ cup **pure maple syrup**

INSTRUCTIONS
1. **Centers:** Put coconut in high-speed blender and blend until it is very fine. (Or use a powerful food processor.)
2. Melt the coconut oil and honey together.
3. Add oil and honey to the coconut in the blender and mix until it is a creamy consistency.
4. Form into 1" balls by squishing mixture together firmly. Place on wax-paper lined cookie sheet. Place in fridge or freezer for an hour or more. (You can flatten the balls a bit if you prefer a disc shape.)
5. **Chocolate Coating:** Melt cacao butter in a bain marie (in a bowl over simmering water—don't let bowl touch water). Remove from heat and whisk in cocoa powder and maple syrup until well mixed and smooth.
6. Using two forks or small spoons, dip coconut balls in the melted chocolate and place on a parchment-lined cookie sheet.
7. Return truffles to fridge or freezer to set. Store in sealed container in fridge or freezer. Serve at room temperature.

TIPS
• If you have leftover melted chocolate, drizzle on top of the coated truffles. Or use as dip for pieces of banana or apple—then roll in unsweetened shredded coconut, hemp seeds or crushed nuts.

WAYS YOU CAN ADAPT OR ENHANCE THIS RECIPE
• *Flavour additons:* Consider adding a few drops (to taste) of peppermint oil or extract, vanilla extract, or any flavoured extract, medicine flower extract, or food-grade essential oil, such as strawberry, lemon or orange. Or for a "cloud 9" treat, add 2 T. of your favourite liquer, such as Ouzo, Limoncello, or Grand Marnier.
• For the chocolate coating, you can substitute with semi- or bitter-sweet chocolate (chips or chopped baking chocolate). Simply melt 1 cup (170g) in a bain marie until melted.

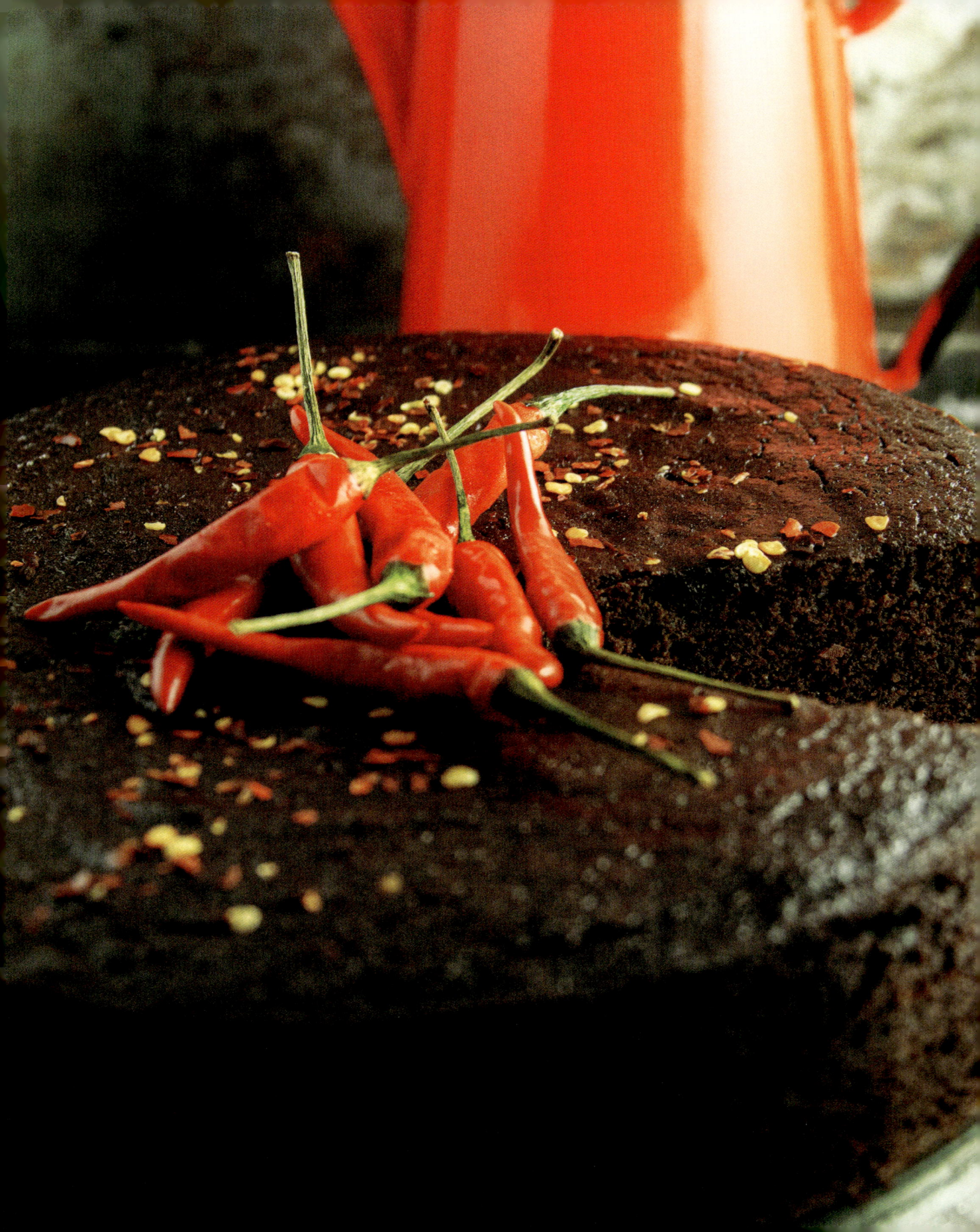

Chocolate & Chili QUINOA CAKE

GF **DF** **NF OPTION**

This reminds me of Mexican Hot Chocolate...rich, creamy chocolate with the spices of cinnamon and chili to give it a little heat that adds flavour to the chocolate. This cake is flourless, gluten-free, grain-free (quinoa is a seed), refined sugar-free, dairy-free, easy to make, and super moist and delicious! (And no one seems to know it's made with quinoa.) Quinoa contains plenty of protein, minerals and B vitamins. The Chocolate-Chili Ganache is basically a chocolate sauce type of topping/icing that's simple and easy to make on the stovetop in five minutes. All so yummy and chocolatey with a subtle spicy bite. *(Or you can frost with Sugarless Chocolate Frosting p.136 , if you prefer.)*

Makes one 9-10" spring-form pan *(or two 8" round pans)*

INGREDIENTS

⅔ cup **quinoa** *(or 2 cups cooked)*
1 ⅓ cups **water**
¾ cup **mild-tasting oil** *(I like avocado oil)*
⅓ cup **almond milk** *(for NF: use Oat Milk, p.149, or coconut milk)*
4 **large eggs**
1 tsp. **pure vanilla extract**
⅓ cup **pure maple syrup** *(or honey or coconut nectar)*
1 cup **coconut sugar**
1 cup **raw cacao powder** *(preferably raw, organic)*
1½ tsp. **baking powder**
½ tsp. **baking soda**
½ tsp. **salt**
1½ tsp. each of **ancho chili powder & cinnamon**
½ tsp. **cayenne** *(use half the amount, if you prefer less heat)*
¼ tsp. **nutmeg**

Double recipe of Chocolate-Chili Ganache (p.136)

INSTRUCTIONS

1. Precook quinoa: Bring quinoa and water to boil in medium saucepan, then reduce to simmer. Cover with a tight-fitting lid, and cook for 12 minutes. Turn heat off, place a piece of paper towel over the saucepan and place the lid back on. Let sit for another 8-10 minutes. Take lid off, fluff with fork, and let cool.
2. Preheat oven to 350° F.
3. Grease 9" spring-form pan liberally with coconut oil. (Optional: Also line bottoms of the pan[s] with parchment paper.)
4. In a blender, combine oil, milk, eggs, vanilla and maple syrup and process briefly. Add the cooled, cooked quinoa. Blend until smooth and creamy.
5. In a large bowl, stir together coconut sugar, cacao powder, baking powder, baking soda, salt and spices. Be sure mixture has no lumps.
6. Add blender contents to the bowl. Stir until well combined.
7. Spread into prepared pan(s). Bake 50-60 minutes, or until done, or until knife or toothpick inserted in center comes out clean. (If baking two 8" pans, bake 40-45 minutes.) Cover with loose foil tent last 10-15 minutes if your cake browns too quickly.
8. Remove from oven and let pan cool on rack. When cool, remove cake from pan. Glaze with room temperature Chocolate-Chili Ganache, or slice cake first and drizzle each piece with warm Chocolate-Chili Ganache. If stacking two round cakes, you can add Chocolate-Chili Ganache between layers.
9. This cake is good served at room temperature, or slightly warm (re-heat 20-30 minutes in 160° F. oven, if necessary).
10. Store in sealed container in fridge for up to a week. Freeze cake without ganache for up to a month—wrap and seal well.

Chocolate Espresso PÂTÉ

GF DF NF EF V P

If you love chocolate and coffee...this is for you! This is a very decadent, rich and creamy chocolate ganache dessert that will please your palate and those of your dinner guests. Serve at your next dinner party and be sure to garnish (see suggestions below). For another impressive treat, serve in Mini Chocolate Cups (p.120) and top with a whole espresso bean. It's also a great make-ahead dessert that can be made a day or two beforehand. This recipe can be made without espresso for a pure "chocolate pâté". Please note that this pâté is a softer, creamier dessert, and, when left at room temperature for awhile, can even be spread on things such as toast, bagels and scones. Or try on Grandad's Oatmeal Cookies (p.35), Flourless Chocolate Cake (p.86) or Flourless Chocolate Cupcakes (p.45), or on fresh fruit such as sliced bananas and apples. My favourite is spread on a baguette (sometimes with a slice of cheese) and served with red wine! Or eat as is—just slice and enjoy with a cup of coffee! Be sure to check out the firmer version of this recipe on the next page—the Chocolate Espresso Ganache Tart.

Serves 8-10   Makes one 7x3" or 8x4" loaf pan

INGREDIENTS

1 cup **full-fat coconut milk** (use all the coconut cream from the can, then top up with milk —see Tips on next page)

1½ T. *(12g)* **cacao butter**, finely chopped

2 T. **pure maple syrup** (or honey or coconut nectar)

1 T. **fresh espresso or coffee beans**, finely ground to powder (can use decaffeinated beans)

1 tsp. **pure vanilla extract** (or ½ tsp. vanilla powder, or scrape inside of ¼ fresh vanilla bean)

¼ tsp. **sea salt**

6 oz. *(170 g)* **good quality bittersweet chocolate** *(70-85% cacao)*, finely chopped.

INSTRUCTIONS

1. Heat coconut milk in saucepan over medium-low heat for a few minutes. (Do not boil.)
2. Stir in the cacao butter, maple syrup, espresso and salt until all ingredients are melted, about 6-8 minutes. Be sure this mixture is hot, but not boiling.
3. Chop the chocolate finely and place in a large bowl along with the vanilla.
4. Pour the hot coconut milk mixture over it, then immediately stir or whisk the mixture until smooth and creamy. (Pour mixture through a fine sieve into chocolate if you prefer no tiny bits of coffee and milder flavour.)
5. Let this ganache mixture sit in the bowl at room temperature for 20-25 minutes, whisking occasionally.
6. Line bottom and sides of loaf pan with two perpendicular flaps of plastic wrap or parchment paper with overhangs to make four "handles" for easier removal later.
7. Pour the cooled mixture into mold (prepared loaf pan).
8. Refrigerate at least 2 hours before serving. Slice and plate with garnish, if desired. (See next page for ideas.)
9. Wrap in plastic and store in fridge for up to 2 weeks.

SEE NEXT PAGE FOR:
- TIPS
- WAYS YOU CAN ADAPT OR ENHANCE THIS RECIPE
- GARNISH AND SERVING IDEAS

Chocolate Espresso GANACHE TART

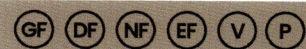

This is the same recipe as previous page *(Chocolate Espresso Pâté)*, but results in a firmer type of ganache, more like a crustless tart or creamy fudge that holds its shape at room temperature.

You just need to add double the chocolate to the previous recipe:
Instead of 6 oz *(170g)* of chocolate, use 12 oz. *(340g)* of chocolate.

TIPS
- *Refrigerate a can of full-fat coconut milk; the coconut cream solidifies and makes it easier to remove. (Save the remaining liquid for smoothies or lattés!) Always keep a can of full-fat coconut milk in the fridge.*
- *My favourite coconut milk is Whole Foods 365 Organic (which contains a good amount of cream). Also good are Native Forest and Thai Kitchen organic coconut milks.*
- *Purchase fresh and quality coffee beans. Grinding coffee beans yourself in a coffee grinder just before use will result in the best flavour. You can, however, substitute with 2 tsp. instant espresso or brewed espresso (or very strong coffee) if needed.*
- *If spreading the paté on something, let sit at room temperature 20 minutes or longer—until desired softness.*

WAYS YOU CAN ADAPT OR ENHANCE THIS RECIPE
- *Substitute espresso in this recipe with 2 tsp. of your favourite liqueur (such as coffee, raspberry, cherry, almond) or bourbon, whiskey or rum.*
- *For refined sugar-free chocolate: Substitute bittersweet chocolate with unsweetened chocolate; then increase your maple syrup to ⅓ - ½ cup and add 1 tsp. of butter, homemade ghee, vegan butter or coconut oil to melted chocolate.*

GARNISH AND SERVING IDEAS
- *Espresso or coffee beans (whole or smashed), or cacao powder (sifted onto dessert and serving plate).*
- *Roasted and chopped nuts, such as pecans, almonds, hazelnuts, pistachios or macadamias.*
- *Fresh raspberries, or berries of choice, or Raspberry Coulis (or coulis using other fruit choices) (p.142).*
- *Coconut whipped cream and topped with shaved chocolate or edible flowers.*
- *A small amount of white or milk chocolate, melted and drizzled on top of each serving.*
- *Cut into squares, then cut through diagonally to make triangle pieces. Or spoon into quenelles and plate with fresh fruit.*

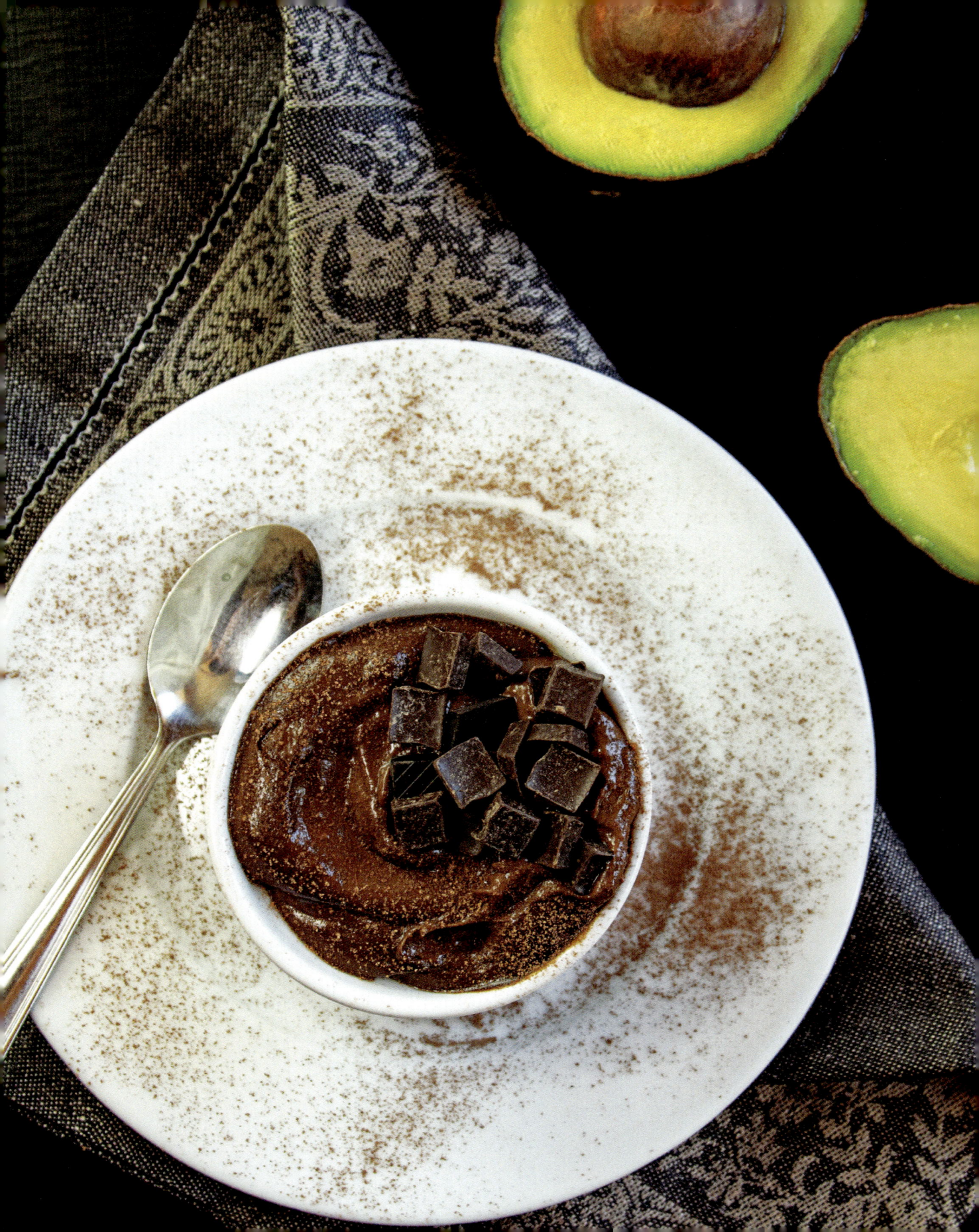

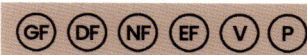

OMG! CHOCOLATE AVOCADO PUDDINGS

OMG! Need I say more? This delicious and creamy pudding is not only versatile, but very healthy! If you love chocolate, you'll love this. And no one can ever tell there's avocado in it! I highly recommend you try out all the flavour variations...they are all OMG delicious! My favourite is the peanut butter. Who doesn't like peanut butter and chocolate? Hellooo! And...get this, you can make the most authentic-tasting Fudgsicles using this recipe (see p.107).

6-8 servings

INGREDIENTS

2 large, or 3 small **ripe avocados**
½ cup **dates**, chopped, pits removed *(soaked in ½ cup hot water for 20 minutes...keep and use water!)*
½ cup **pure maple syrup** *(or more, to taste)*
¾ cup **cacao powder** *(preferably raw, organic)*
14-oz. can **full-fat coconut milk**
1 tsp. **pure vanilla extract**
pinch **sea salt**

INSTRUCTIONS

1. Place all ingredients in food processor or blender (including the saved water). Blend until smooth.
2. Serve immediately or pour into dessert cups or bowls. Cover with plastic wrap (press plastic down onto pudding so no skin forms). Refrigerate.
3. Optional topping ideas: Before serving you can top each pudding with fresh fruit, coconut whipped cream, chocolate chips, cacao nibs, mint sprigs, toasted coconut, or toasted chopped nuts.

FLAVOUR VARIATIONS

Just add to the above recipe:

- **Chocolate PEANUT BUTTER Pudding:** Add ½ - ⅔ cup peanut butter and ¼ cup honey. *(Contains nuts.)*
- **Chocolate ORANGE Pudding:** Soak the dates in juice of one fresh orange (instead of water) and add zest from that orange to the mixture.
- **Chocolate MINT Pudding:** Add ¼ - ½ tsp. good quality mint extract.
- **Chocolate PISTACHIO Pudding:** Blend in ½ tsp. almond extract. Stir in roughly chopped pistachios and garnish with a few more. *(Contains nuts.)*
- **Chocolate COFFEE Pudding:** Soak the dates in ½ cup very strong coffee or espresso instead of water (and remember to use the soaking water!), or add 1-2 T. coffee beans to the blender.

WAYS YOU CAN ADAPT OR ENHANCE THIS RECIPE

- V options: Replace honey with coconut nectar; and replace butter or ghee with coconut oil or vegan butter.
- For refined sugar-free chocolate coating, use unsweetened chocolate and melt with 2 tsp. of coconut oil or homemade ghee. Remove from heat and whisk in 2 T. maple syrup or honey.
- Any extra melted chocolate you may have can be drizzled over top of the dipped truffles. Or drizzle on melted white or milk chocolate for pretty contrast.
- You can also use this recipe as a fruit dip, as a layer in a Parfait (p.54), or as a filling in Mini Chocolate Cups (p.120).
- Top pudding servings with a dollop of coconut whipped cream, 3 or 4 fresh berries or chocolate chips, and a sprig of mint.

FLOURLESS CHOCOLATE CAKE
with Raspberry Coulis

Chocolate and raspberry together—what's not to love?! If you like mango and chocolate, try the mango coulis indicated in the Raspberry Coulis recipe, (p.142). And be sure to try the Whiskey Caramel Sauce and Sugarless Chocolate Frosting versions below.

Makes one 9-10" spring-form pan (or two 8" round pans)

INGREDIENTS

⅔ cup **dry quinoa** (or 2 cups cooked)
1⅓ cups **water**
¾ cup **mild-tasting oil** (I like avocado oil)
⅓ cup **almond milk** (for NF: use Oat Milk, p.149 or coconut milk)
4 large **eggs**
1 tsp. **pure vanilla extract**
⅓ cup **pure maple syrup** (or honey or coconut nectar)
1 cup **coconut sugar**
1 cup **cacao powder** (preferably raw, organic)
1½ tsp. **baking powder**
½ tsp. **baking soda**
½ tsp. **salt**

One recipe of Raspberry Coulis (p.142).

with Whiskey Caramel Sauce
Follow cake recipe above, but instead of serving with Raspberry Coulis, serve with a Whiskey Caramel Sauce. Follow recipe for Boozy Caramel Sauce (p.133). For a "salted" Whiskey Caramel Sauce, sprinkle caramel sauce with a pinch of flaked sea salt right before serving.

with Sugarless Chocolate Frosting
Follow cake recipe above, but instead of serving with Raspberry Coulis, frost the cake with Sugarless Chocolate Frosting (p.136).

INSTRUCTIONS

1. Precook quinoa: Bring quinoa and water to boil in medium saucepan, then reduce to simmer.
Cover with a tight-fitting lid, and cook for 12 minutes. Turn heat off, place a piece of paper towel over the saucepan and place the lid back on. Let sit for another 8-10 minutes. Take lid off, fluff with fork, and let cool.
2. Preheat oven to 350° F.
3. Grease 9" springform pan liberally with coconut oil. (Optional: Also line bottoms of the pan[s] with parchment paper.)
4. In a blender, combine oil, milk, eggs, vanilla and maple syrup and process briefly. Add the cooled, cooked quinoa. Blend until smooth and creamy.
5. In a large bowl, stir together sugar, cacao powder, baking powder, baking soda and salt. Be sure mixture has no lumps.
6. Add blender contents to the bowl. Stir until well combined.
7. Spread into prepared pan(s). Bake 50-60 minutes, or until done, or until knife or toothpick inserted in center comes out clean. (If baking two 8" pans, bake 40-45 minutes.) Cover with loose foil tent last 10-15 minutes if your cake browns too quickly.
8. Remove from oven and let pan cool on rack. When cool, remove cake from pan.
9. Serve each slice of cake with drizzle of Raspberry Coulis.
10. This cake is good served at room temperature, or slightly warm (re-heat 20-30 minutes in 160° F. oven if necessary).
11. Store in sealed container in fridge for up to a week. Freezes well for up to a month.

Dark Chocolate PECAN CLUSTERS
WITH SEA SALT

(GF) (DF) (EF) (V) (P)

Just 3 ingredients! A very easy and quick recipe. Good source of protein and antioxidants. Great served with coffee or wine, or a healthy afternoon pick-me-up. Or serve as a small treat after a meal. You can substitute pecans with other nuts. (See adaptation below.) Try to find good quality chocolate that is 70-85% of pure cacao for better nutrition (fibre, potassium, magnesium, calcium, copper and of course antioxidants). The less milk and sugar the chocolate contains, the better. See refined sugar-free option below using unsweetened chocolate (adding your own healthy sweetener).

INGREDIENTS

2-2½ cups **raw pecan halves** *(see Adaptations below)*
8 oz. *(225g)* **bittersweet chocolate** *(70-85% cacao)*, chopped *(see Adaptations)*
flaked sea salt or fleur de sel *(see Adaptations)*

WAYS YOU CAN ADAPT OR ENHANCE THIS RECIPE

- *Substitute pecans with other nuts, such as almonds, hazelnuts, Brazil nuts or walnuts. (Roasting times may vary.)*
- *For refined sugar-free chocolate, use unsweetened baking chocolate and melt with 2 tsp. of virgin coconut oil, homemade ghee, or vegan butter. Then whisk in 2 T. pure maple syrup or honey.*
- *Top with fleur de sel, flaked sea salt (such as Maldon), coarse sea salt, or flavoured sea salts, such as smoked, vanilla or ancho chili. For a low-salt diet, replace salt with a few sprinkles of hemp seeds, coconut, or toasted pumpkin or sesame seeds.*
- *For a "turtle" cluster, simply drizzle with warm Caramel Sauce (p.131) over chilled/set chocolates and return to fridge to set. For salted caramel, add a pinch of flaked sea salt or fleur de sel.*
- *For Nut & Fruit Chocolate Clusters, add ¼ cup chopped, dried fruit (such as cherries, apricots, cranberries, mulberries or figs) to step #4 in instructions.*

INSTRUCTIONS

1. Preheat oven to 300° F.
2. Spread pecan halves on baking pan in single layer and roast for 10-12 minutes. Stir once or twice during this time to ensure even toasting. (Watch closely—they can burn quickly.) Remove from oven and let cool.
3. Slowly melt chocolate in a double boiler, or in a bowl over simmering water until melted. Remove from heat.
4. Add roasted pecans to chocolate and stir to coat.
5. Spoon clusters onto a parchment or waxed paper lined cookie sheet.
6. Wait 5 minutes and then pinch a few granules of flaked or coarse sea salt on top of each cluster, to taste. (See salt options provided.)
7. Place tray of clusters in fridge until set, about 30 minutes.
8. These keep well! Store in sealed container in the fridge for up to a month.

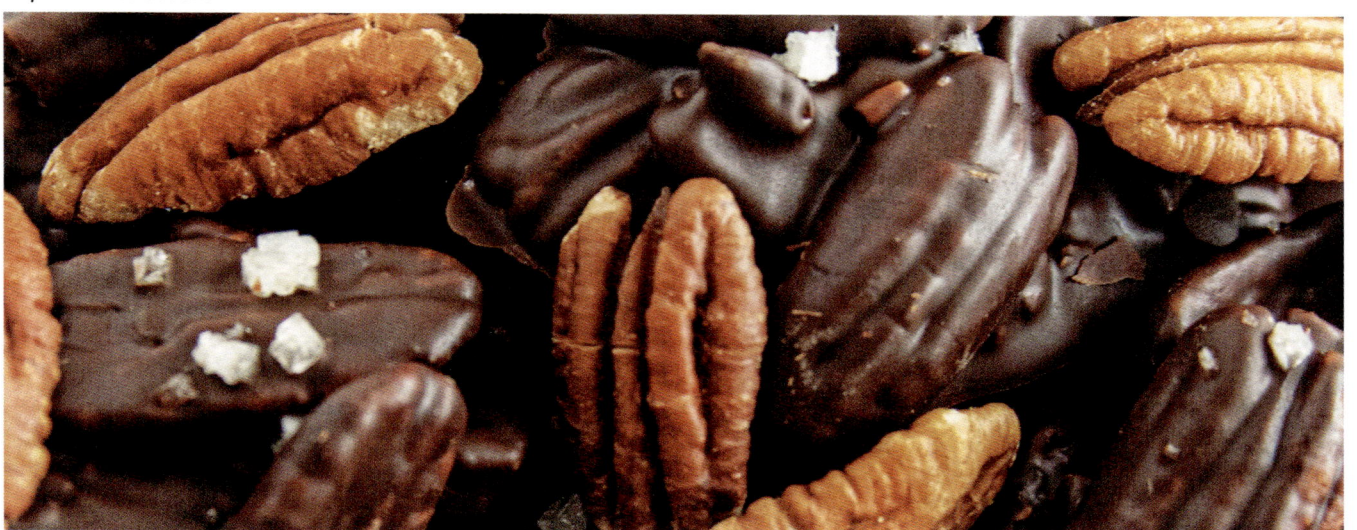

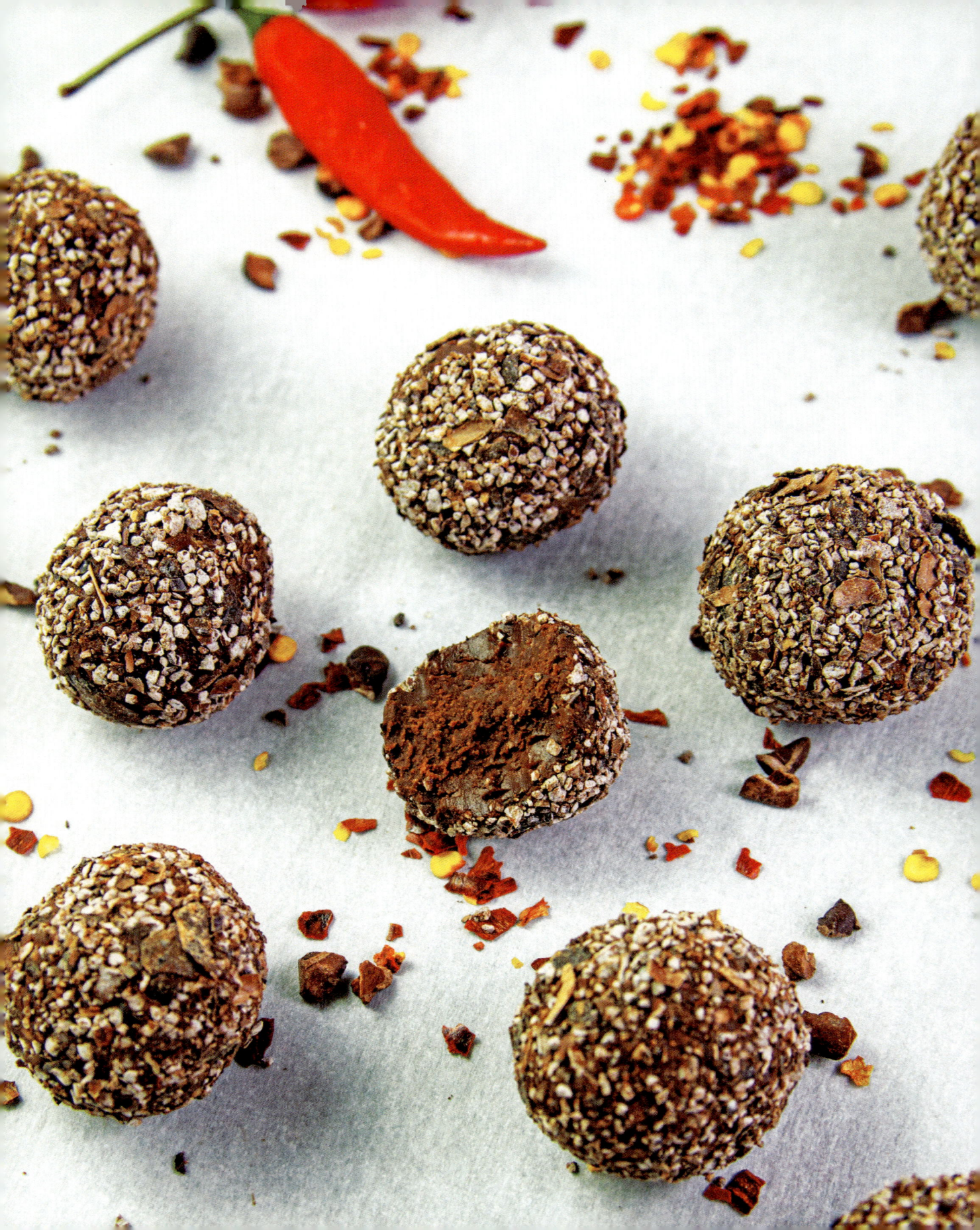

Chocolate CHEVRE TRUFFLES

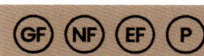

3 WAYS

These delicious truffles are smooth and flavourful. The goat cheese pairs well with the chocolate—this is an amazing culinary combination. These truffles are surprisingly tasty and most people don't even know there is any cheese in them! If you like lemon and you like chocolate, you'll love these. If you like the combination of spicy chili pepper and chocolate, you'll love the variations below. My family likes all three versions, that's why you're getting all three!

CHOCOLATE & LEMON CHEVRE TRUFFLES

4 oz. *(120g)* **unsweetened chocolate**, chopped
½ cup **honey** *(preferably raw, organic) (or coconut nectar or pure maple syrup)*
½ packed cup *(4 oz./120g)* **chevre** *(soft goat cheese)*, room temperature
½ tsp. **pure vanilla extract**
½ tsp. **pure lemon extract** *(or a few drops of food-grade lemon essential oil, to taste)*
pinch **sea salt**
For Rolling: approx. ¼ cup **raw cacao powder** *(or ground cacao nibs)*

MEXICAN HOT CHOCOLATE TRUFFLES *(Think France meets Mexico!)*

Follow the ingredients and instructions for lemon truffles, but omit the lemon extract, and instead add ½ tsp. each of ancho chili powder and cinnamon, ⅛ tsp. each of cayenne, black pepper and nutmeg. Optional: Add 2-3 T. of cacao nibs or 2 T. of pecan butter (or ground pecans). Garnish with chili flakes.

CHOCOLATE & CHILI CHEVRE TRUFFLES *(Pictured)*

Follow the ingredients and instructions above, but simply omit the lemon extract, and instead add ½ tsp. red chili pepper flakes, and ¼ tsp. each of ground black pepper & cayenne (to taste).
Optional: Add 1-2 T. roughly ground coffee beans for a "chocolate-chili-coffee" version. Garnish with chili flakes or coffee bean.

INSTRUCTIONS

1. Melt chocolate in a bain marie (in a bowl over a pot of simmering water—do not let bowl touch water) until melted.
2. Remove from heat and whisk in the rest of the ingredients (except the cacao powder) until well blended and smooth.
3. Cover bowl and place in fridge for 1 hour to harden.
4. Roll into 1" balls, then roll in cacao powder. (Optional: Garnish with lemon zest.)
5. Refrigerate in sealed container for up to 2 weeks. (Note: Best served at room temperature. Let sit out 30 minutes.)

TIPS

• *Use good quality extracts for best flavour. I use "Simply Organic" brand. Or use food-grade essential oils, but be sure to start with just 1 or 2 drops and taste after each added drop. Medicine flower extracts are also a good option.*
• *Check honey resource on p. 12 for delicious, mild-tasting, creamy raw honey. It's 100% pure Canadian, well-priced, and they deliver.*

WAYS YOU CAN ADAPT OR ENHANCE THIS RECIPE

• *Two more delicious flavour variations (to replace lemon extract): strawberry extract (or medicine flower extract), or licorice-flavoured liqueur (such as Ouzo, Pernod or Absinthe). If using liqueurs to flavour these truffles, be sure to add 2-3 T., or to taste.*

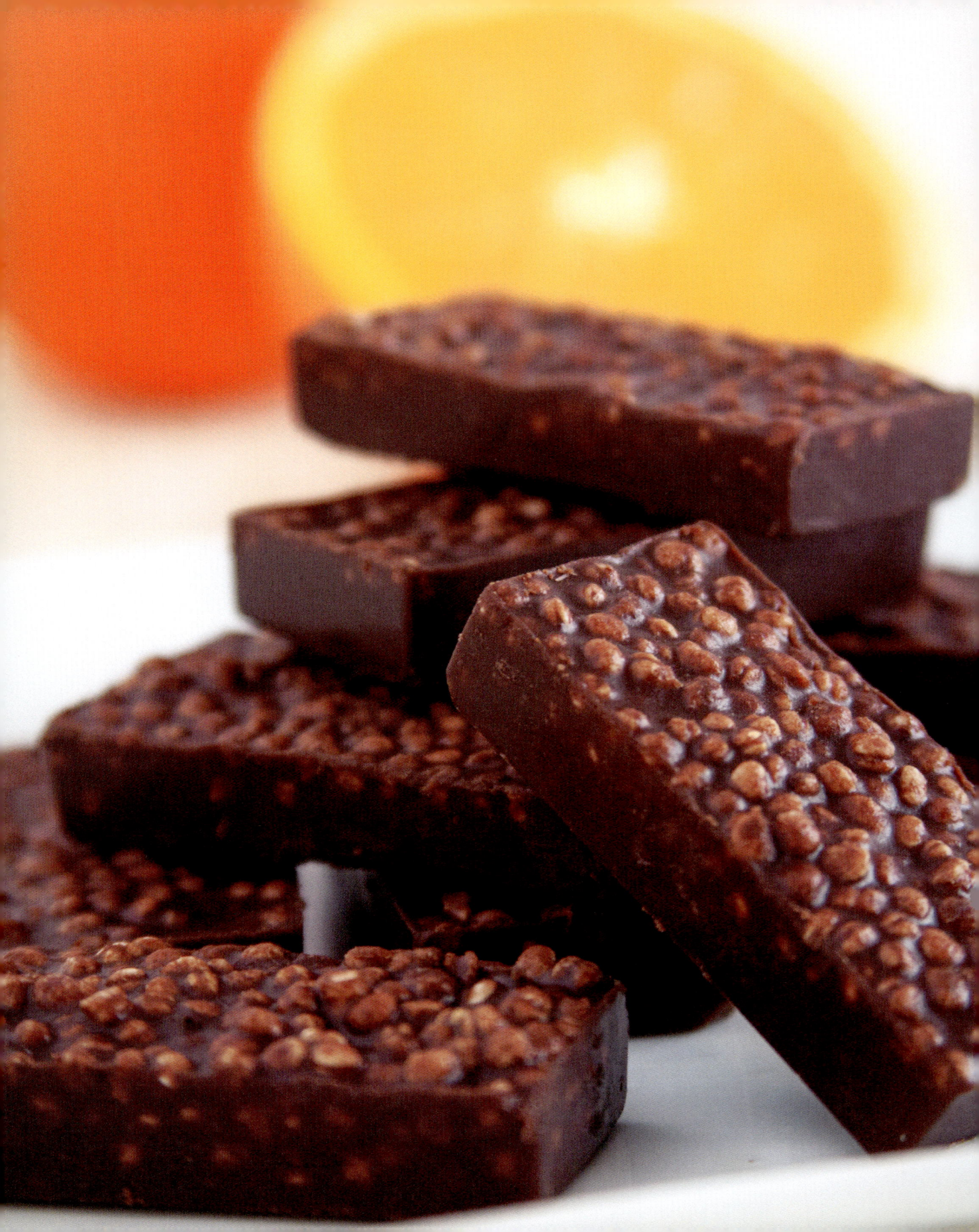

Crunchy CHOCOLATE BITES

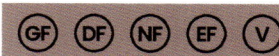

Oh, so chocolatey and crunchy! These little chocolate bars fill the chocolate craving and sweet spot…and no guilt…these babies are good for you! Loaded with protein, antioxidants, fibre and healthy fats. I like them for breakfast with coffee. (Okay, I admit, I'm addicted to these.) They also make a great afternoon pick-me-up. Kids of all ages like these—they are like little guiltless chocolate bars. And so easy to make. This is definitely worth getting the ingredients to make! I've included here my five favourite flavour combinations.
Make in heart molds for Valentine's Day.

INGREDIENTS

¾ cup **cacao butter** *(95 g or 3.3 oz.—approx. ⅔ cup)*, chopped

¼ cup **virgin coconut oil**

½ tsp. **pure vanilla extract**

⅓ cup **pure maple syrup** *(or honey or coconut nectar)*

1 cup **cacao powder** *(preferably raw, organic)*, sifted to remove any lumps

¼ cup **cacao nibs**

¼ cup **puffed quinoa** *(cereal)*

⅓ cup **"Buckwheat Crunchies"** *(see Tips)*, **or organic crispy rice cereal**

INSTRUCTIONS

1. Place the cacao butter and coconut oil in a bain marie (in a medium-sized bowl over a pot of simmering water—the bowl should not touch the water) until melted.
2. Remove bowl from heat and whisk in the vanilla, maple syrup and cacao powder.
3. Stir in the cacao nibs, puffed quinoa and buckwheat crunchies.
4. Spoon into silicone molds or paper-lined mini muffin cups. (See notes for topping ideas.)
5. Refrigerate until set 1-2 hours. Pop out of molds and serve.
6. These stay well at room temperature for a short period of time, but best to keep stored in sealed container in fridge for up to 2 weeks.

TIPS

• Buckwheat Crunchies are soaked and dehydrated raw buckwheat groats, dried until they are crunchy. Feel free to substitute Buckwheat Crunchies with crispy rice cereal or more puffed quinoa. This recipe is flexible that way. (Surprisingly, buckwheat is NOT a wheat—it is actually a fruit seed and is highly nutritious, gluten-free, has a high content of protein and fibre, significant amounts of iron, phosphorus, copper, zinc, manganese and magnesium and is a good source of linoleic fatty acids and B vitamins. It contains all 8 essential amino acids and is packed with phytonutrients and antioxidants.)
• Get good quality extracts—they make a difference. I use "Simply Organic" brand of mint and orange extracts. Consider trying different flavour extracts, such as coffee, cherry or strawberry. Or search for medicine flower extracts.

WAYS YOU CAN ADAPT OR ENHANCE THIS RECIPE

• *Chocolate Orange (pictured)* – Add ½ tsp. orange extract to step #2 above.
• *Mint Chocolate (pictured on front cover)* – Add ½ tsp. mint extract to step #2 above.
• *Espresso Lemon* – Add 1 T. finely ground coffee beans (or 1-2 tsp. instant espresso powder) and ½ tsp. lemon extract. (Can use decaffeinated coffee beans.)
• *Almond* – Omit crispy puffed quinoa and crispy rice cereal and instead add ½ - ¾ cup chopped, raw or roasted almonds to step #3 above. In place of roasted almonds, try roasted hazelnuts, pistachios, brazil nuts, macadamias, pecans or pumpkin seeds.
• *Chipotle Cardamom Cinnamon* – Add 1 tsp. each ground chipotle, cardamom and cinnamon to step #2 above.
• *Topping ideas:* sprinkle each bite with a pinch puffed quinoa, fleur de sel or flaked sea salt, cacao nibs, chopped/roasted nuts or smashed coffee beans just before refrigerating.

BREAKFASTS & BEVERAGES

BREAKFASTS

Dutch Apple Pancakes *93*

Turmeric & Spice Millet Breakfast Bowl *94*

Easy Nutty Granola *95*

Gluten-Free Banana Muffins *96*

Blackberry & Lemon Clafouti *97*

BEVERAGES

Lattés & Frappés *98-99*

Mexican Chili & Cinnamon Hot Chocolate *100*

Orange Julia *101*

Citrus Martini *101*

Ginger & Turmeric Hot Beverage *and* Iced Frappé *102*

Dutch APPLE PANCAKES

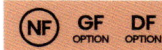

This is impressive visually, and absolutely delicious. A family favourite, especially on weekends. It's always a hit with breakfast and brunch guests. If you tolerate dairy, try this recipe with butter (grass-fed or organic) since it makes for a nice flavour.

IMPORTANT NOTE: **This makes one large pancake, which is 1 serving**. Simply multiply the recipe by the number of servings desired. You will need a pie plate (preferably nonstick) for each pancake!
(If you don't have enough pie plates on hand, you can purchase inexpensive aluminum foil pie pans.)

TOPPING

1 **apple**
1 T. **grass-fed butter**, melted and cooled *(for DF: use coconut oil or vegan butter)*
2 T. pure **maple syrup**
1 tsp. **cinnamon**

PANCAKES

¼ cup **spelt flour** *(or white flour, GF all-purpose flour mix, or flour of your choice)*
¼ tsp. **sea salt**
¼ cup **milk of choice** *(i.e. coconut milk, nut milk)*
2 **eggs**
2 T. **grass-fed butter**, for pie pan *(for DF: use coconut oil or vegan butter)*

TOPPING INSTRUCTIONS

DO AHEAD: 1. Preheat oven to 425° F.
2. 1 apple, pared, cored and sliced. Set aside.
3. Separately, in a small measuring cup, whisk together the 1 T. melted butter, maple syrup and cinnamon. Set aside.

PANCAKES INSTRUCTIONS

4. In 8-cup measuring cup or large bowl, whisk together flour, salt and milk until well combined.
5. Whisk in 1 egg at a time, whisking thoroughly before adding the next egg.
6. When oven is preheated and topping and pancake batter are ready to go, then place 2 T. butter in (each) 8" pie plate. Place in preheated oven for about 2 minutes, or until butter melts and starts to bubble.

ASSEMBLY INSTRUCTIONS

Important: Work quickly for this next part so pie plate does not cool!
7. Remove pie plate from oven and swirl butter to coat bottom of pie plate.
8. Quickly pour egg mixture into pie pan, sprinkle apple pieces on top, then pour maple-cinnamon mixture on top.
9. Immediately return pie plate to oven and bake 18 minutes.
10. Remove from oven and carefully transfer the pancake onto a serving plate. Serve immediately. (Optional: Serve with drizzle of maple syrup and/or a dollop of Thick Cashew Cream, p. 148)

TIPS

- *Note: Different flours all result in a slightly different taste and texture.*

Turmeric & Spice MILLET BREAKFAST BOWL

I had fun creating this and it is one of my favourite breakfasts in the winter. It's hearty, warming, flavourful, and just the right combination of soft, crunchy, savory, sweet and spicy. I could easily have called this recipe "Anti-Inflammatory Breakfast Bowl". With the selected ingredients, it's highly anti-inflammatory. Turmeric and ginger are particularly known for their anti-inflammatory properties. The fat in the pumpkin seeds and coconut milk are anti-inflammatory. Millet is one of the best choices for an anti-inflammatory grain; it is an ancient grain packed with calcium, protein, iron, potassium, B vitamins and dietary fibre. Consider adding extra anti-inflammatory and nutritious toppings (listed below). Feel free to play with the spices and ingredients in this basic recipe to suit your individual taste—the quantities and ingredients listed are flexible.

Serves 1 (Simply multiply by number of servings you wish to make.)

INGREDIENTS

1 cup **cooked millet** *(See alternate grains below)*
¼ - ⅓ cup **coconut milk** *(or almond milk)*
¼ - ½ tsp. **turmeric** *(to taste)*
½ tsp. each of **cinnamon,** and **ginger**
¼ tsp. each of **cardamom, nutmeg, allspice**
⅛ tsp. **black pepper** *(see Tips)*
Splash of **almond milk** *(for NF: see adaptations)*
½ **banana**, sliced
2 T. pure **maple syrup** *(or coconut nectar, or
1 T. melted honey)*
1 T. each **pistachios, pumpkin seeds** and **walnuts** *(for NF: see Adaptations)*
1 T. dried **goji berries** or **dried cranberries** *(or fresh or dried fruit of choice)*

INSTRUCTIONS

1. Heat cooked millet, coconut milk and spices in a small saucepan until heated through. Add a little water, if necessary.
2. Remove from heat and transfer mixture to a bowl. Add in the following order: almond milk, banana, maple syrup, nuts & seeds, fruit. Enjoy warm!

TIPS
• When using turmeric, always be sure to add black pepper because it activates the anti-inflammatory properties of turmeric to make it bio-available. Consider adding freshly grated ginger into the mix for even more anti-inflammatory benefits.

WAYS YOU CAN ADAPT OR ENHANCE THIS RECIPE
• My favourite grain for this breakfast bowl is millet; however, you can also use other cooked whole grains such as quinoa, amaranth, sorghum, buckwheat and rice.
• For NF: use seeds only (pumpkin, sunflower, hemp, etc.) and substitute almond milk with Oat Milk (p.149).
• Consider adding these anti-inflammatory and nutritious toppings: Flax, chia, hemp or sunflower seeds, almonds or walnuts, Buckwheat Crunchies (see notes on p.91), or fresh berries.

Easy
NUTTY GRANOLA

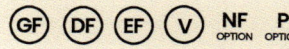

It took a few tries to create a delicious but super easy granola recipe. This is it! It is loaded with protein and nutrition. A great way to start the day! Enjoy it with Almond Milk (p.147) (or other nut milk), Cashew Milk (p.148), or Oat Milk (p. 149) and some fresh sliced banana or fresh berries.

INGREDIENTS

6-6½ cups **rolls oats** *(use gluten-free, if desired)*
3-4 cups **nuts & seeds** of choice *(I use pecans, walnuts, brazil nuts, almonds, hazelnuts, pumpkin seeds, sunflower seeds & sesame seeds)*
2-3 cups **coconut flakes** *(also called coconut ribbons or chips)*
1 cup **avocado oil** *(or other mild-tasting oil)*
1 cup **pure maple syrup**
1 T. **pure vanilla extract**
2 pinches **sea salt**
1-2 cups **dried fruit** of choice *(cranberries, cherries, mulberries, goji berries, etc.)*, optional

INSTRUCTIONS

1. Preheat oven to 325° F.
2. Place rolls oats, nuts & seeds, and coconut in large bowl and mix to blend.
3. Place avocado oil, maple syrup, vanilla and sea salt in small bowl and whisk until blended.
4. Pour liquid mixture over dry mixture and stir well to coat all ingredients.
5. Spread mixture onto 2 extra-large parchment-lined baking sheets.
6. Place in preheated oven for 30 minutes, stirring every 10 minutes.
7. Turn oven off and let sit for another 10 minutes.
8. Open oven door and let sit for 30 minutes to dry out.
9. When granola is cool, add dried fruit and stir to mix.
10. Store in sealed containers, such as large canning jars. (Keeps well in fridge or freezer.)

WAYS YOU CAN ADAPT OR ENHANCE THIS RECIPE
• Paleo option: Omit rolled oats and increase nuts and seeds to 8-9 cups. Increase coconut flakes to 4 cups.
• NF option: Omit nuts and increase amount of seeds and coconut flakes.

Gluten Free BANANA MUFFINS

It's so great to have a recipe that uses up overripe bananas! (Be sure to use bananas that are soft and have brown spots.) These healthy muffins are quick and easy to make. Sorghum flour is an ancient grain and contains a nutritional punch with an abundance of vitamins, minerals, antioxidants and protein (as much protein as quinoa!). It contains a high amount of dietary fibre, is slow to digest, and helps with blood sugar balancing. I highly recommend using sorghum flour for this recipe.
I particularly like these warm shortly after taking out of the oven. The next day I like to toast them in my toaster oven and then spread on some almond butter, grass-fed butter or No-Cook Fruit Jam (p.146).

Makes 10-12 muffins

INGREDIENTS

1 cup + 2 T. **sorghum flour** *(or GF all-purpose flour mix; or half cup + 1 T. of each)*
1½ tsp. **baking powder**
½ tsp. **baking soda**
⅔ cup **coconut sugar**
1 - 1½ tsp. **mace** *(or other spice such as cinnamon, allspice, cardamom or ginger)*, optional
pinch **sea salt**
2 **large eggs**
⅔ cup **avocado oil**, or other neutral tasting oil
⅓ cup **milk** of choice *(such as almond, oat, cashew)*
1¼ cups **overripe bananas** *(about 4 bananas)*, mashed well *(see Tips)*
Optional Topping:
20-30 **raw almonds**, roughly chopped or left whole

INSTRUCTIONS

1. Preheat oven to 400° F.
2. Grease muffin pan with coconut oil, or line with muffin liners.
3. Sift flour into a large bowl. Stir in baking powder, baking soda, coconut sugar, mace and salt to combine.
4. In a medium-sized bowl, beat together eggs and oil. Add milk and mashed bananas and beat until well combined.
5. Gently stir the wet mixture into the dry mixture. Stir until just combined—do not overmix.
6. Scoop about ⅓ cup into each lined muffin cups. Sprinkle with almonds, if using.
7. Bake 17-18 minutes, or until toothpick inserted in middle comes out clean.
8. Remove from oven, cool for 3-5 minutes, then invert onto baking rack to cool further.
9. Store in sealed container for 3 or 4 days.

TIPS
• Only use overripe bananas—they should be soft and covered with brown spots. Mash well with a fork in a shallow bowl, then measure—do not use more than 1½ cups or muffins may not cook in middle.

WAYS YOU CAN ADAPT OR ENHANCE THIS RECIPE
• Optional: Top each muffin with a sprinkle of any nuts or seeds.

Blackberry and Lemon CLAFOUTI

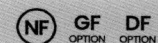

Clafouti is a French fruit pancake baked in the oven, and traditionally made with black cherries, but here I have combined blackberries and lemon zest to create a delicious new version. Several fruit options are listed below. It's healthy, easy and quick to make, and only takes 20 minutes to bake.

IMPORTANT NOTE: *This* **makes one large pancake**, *which is 1 serving.* Simply multiply the recipe by the number of servings. You will need a pie plate (preferably non-stick) for each pancake! (If you don't have enough pie plates on hand, you can purchase inexpensive aluminum foil pie pans.)

INGREDIENTS

1-1½ cups **frozen blackberries**, thawed & drained *(or ¾-1 cup fresh blackberries)*
2 **eggs**, room temperature
½ cup **coconut milk**, room temperature *(or nut milk, or any milk of choice)*
2 T. **butter** *(for pie pan) (for DF: use vegan butter or coconut oil)*
¼ cup **spelt flour** *(or white flour) (for GF: use GF all-purpose flour mix)*
1 packed tsp. **lemon zest**
¼ tsp. **sea salt**
2 T. **pure maple syrup** *(or honey or coconut nectar)*
¾ tsp. **pure vanilla**

INSTRUCTIONS

DO AHEAD:
1. If using frozen berries, thaw and drain.
2. Set eggs and coconut milk out.
3. Preheat oven to 400° F.
4. Place butter in (each) 8" pie plate.
5. Whisk eggs in large bowl until well beaten. Continue whisking adding one ingredient at a time: the milk, flour, lemon zest, salt, maple syrup and vanilla.
6. Place pie plate with butter in preheated oven for about 2-3 minutes, or until butter melts and starts to bubble.

ASSEMBLY:

Important: Work quickly for this next part so pie plate does not cool!
7. Remove pie plate from oven and swirl butter to coat bottom.
8. Quickly pour egg mixture into pie pan, then sprinkle blackberries on top.
9. Immediately return pie plate to oven and bake 20-23 minutes, or until centre puffs up.
10. Remove from oven and carefully transfer the pancake onto a serving plate and serve while it's hot.

WAYS YOU CAN ADAPT OR ENHANCE THIS RECIPE

- *Substitute blackberries with any berry (blueberries, raspberries, strawberries), stone fruits (pitted cherry halves, sliced peaches, nectarines, plums, apricots or prunes), or sliced apples or pears.*
- *Serve with drizzle of maple syrup and/or a dollop of Thick Cashew Cream (p.148) or plain Greek yogurt and some freshly grated lemon zest.*

LATTÉS & FRAPPÉS

Use milks of choice to create these delicious lattés. You can use dairy milk if you choose (although dairy can be inflammatory). I have made recommendations for alternative milk for each latté. If you have an espresso machine, steam these lattés for a nice froth; otherwise heat in a saucepan and use a stick blender to create a froth. For a boozy version, add 1 tsp. of your favorite liquor or liqueur to your latté. (Consider Amaretto, Whiskey or Brandy.) Be sure to try these as Iced Lattés and Frappés (see next page)—they are delicious! My son says the Chocolate Mocha "Iced Latté" is the best he's ever tasted, and he does a lot of take-out coffee drinks.

1. Pumpkin Spice LATTÉ MIX

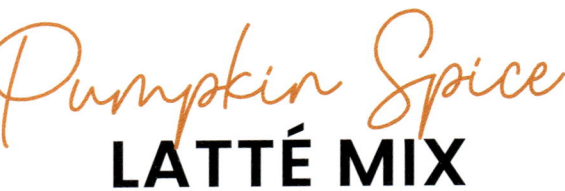
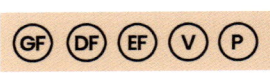

Here is a homemade mix for a Pumpkin Spice Latte. This is so delicious that when I had to be off coffee for awhile (imagine that!), I found it was less difficult by having something so delicious and satisfying to replace it. Consider making your own almond milk and then steam a mug of it with some of this mix. Yum!
Add latté mix to your choice of espresso or coffee and steamed milk—or just add to a steamed milk, hot chocolate, milkshake, iced coffee or smoothie. Make ahead and store in sealed jar in the fridge for up to 10 days.

INGREDIENTS

15-ounce can **pure pumpkin puree** *(pumpkin should be the only ingredient)*
⅓ cup **coconut sugar**
3 T. **pure maple syrup** *(or use more coconut sugar)*
1 T. **pumpkin pie spice** *(or more, to taste) (Make your own — see p.58)*
1½ tsp. **pure vanilla extract**
⅓ cup **almond butter**
Pinch **sea salt**

INSTRUCTIONS

1. Combine all ingredients in a bowl until completely combined.
2. Transfer to a sealed jar or container and store in fridge for up to 2 weeks. Or serve on top of pancakes, toast or ice cream.
3. Add 2-3 T. (or to taste) of mixture to steamed milk or coffee latté of your choice (delicious with homemade Almond Milk. p.147, or coconut milk). Add a shot of espresso, if desired.
4. Optional: Top with coconut whipped cream, a pinch of pumpkin pie spice and poke in a cinnamon stick.

2. Caramel LATTÉ

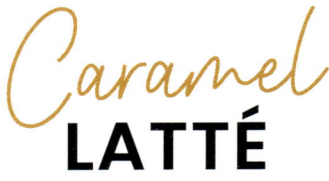
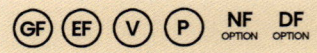

Using Caramel Sauce of your choice (p.131-133), place 1-2 T. into a mug of steamed milk of choice.
Use any alternative milk, but my favourite for this latté is homemade Oat Milk (p.149).
Add a shot or two of espresso or strong coffee, if desired.

3. Chocolate MOCHA LATTÉ

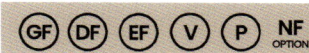

Using Chocolate Chili Ganache (minus the spices) (p.136), Almond Butter Chocolate Sauce (p.135) or Chocolate Sauce of your choice (p.135-136), add 2-3 T. to each mug of hot espresso or coffee and steamed milk.

WAYS YOU CAN ADAPT OR ENHANCE THIS RECIPE
- *Use any alternative milk, but in this case, a creamy milk is best, such as homemade Cashew Milk (p.148), or full-fat coconut milk. Or use combination of coconut milk and almond milk.*
- *Optional: Top with coconut whipped cream and sprinkle with cacao nibs.*
- *For Chocolate "Mint" Mocha, add ¼ tsp. of good quality peppermint extract (and at Christmas, top with coconut whipped cream and sprinkle with red and green Sprinkles, p.125).*

4. Coffee Alternative LATTÉ

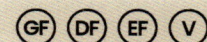

If you ever had to stop drinking coffee, this could be your new go-to drink. It has the texture and body of coffee, but the flavour is different—it's made with dandelion, chicory, beet roots, barley and rye grains. It contains Vitamins A & K (think skin health), and is packed with antioxidants. It does taste different, but that's where this recipe comes in—it's a delicious combination of flavours and I often have it mid-afternoon when I feel like a warm drink but don't want the caffeine.

INGREDIENTS
1¼ cups **Cashew Milk** (p.148) *(or other creamy alternative milk)*
2 tsp. **dandelion herbal beverage powder** *(I use "Dandy Blend")*
½ tsp. **cinnamon**
1-2 tsp. **coconut nectar** *(or pure maple syrup or honey)*
½ tsp. **pure vanilla extract** *(or almond extract)*

INSTRUCTIONS
1. Combine cashew milk, dandelion beverage powder, cinnamon and coconut nectar. Stir well and then steam (or heat and froth).
2. Stir in vanilla and enjoy.
3. Adjust amount of sweetener to your liking.

5. Iced LATTÉS & FRAPPÉS

Iced Latté: Make any of the above lattés and pour over ice.
Frappé: Make any of the above lattés and blend with ice.
You may want to add a little more sweetener. Serve and enjoy immediately.
(See also Ginger & Turmeric Iced Frappé on page 102.)

Mexican Chili & Cinnamon HOT CHOCOLATE

GF DF NF EF V P

I created this recipe kind of by accident. I was making a chocolate-chili ganache for the Chocolate & Chili Quinoa Cake (p.81) and after a photographing session, I had some leftover. I happened to have some coconut milk in the fridge, leftover from a can I opened a few days before, and so I added some coconut milk to the leftover ganache in a pot on the stove and OMG, it was so good. So... it's a keeper! It's a very warming hot chocolate with the added spices. It's rich, so I suggest having a small serving.

Makes 4 small servings

INGREDIENTS

14-oz. can full-fat or light **coconut milk** *(see Adaptations below)*
¼ cup **virgin coconut oil**
¼ cup **cacao powder** *(preferably raw, organic)*
¼ cup **pure maple syrup** *(or honey, coconut nectar or healthy sweetener of choice)*
pinch **sea salt**
¼ tsp. each of **ancho chili powder**, **cinnamon & cayenne** *(use half the cayenne, if you prefer less heat)*
½ tsp. **pure vanilla extract**

INSTRUCTIONS

1. Whisk together all ingredients (except vanilla) together in small saucepan over medium-low heat, whisking while it's heating to blend ingredients.
2. Remove from heat and stir in vanilla. Pour into mugs and enjoy while hot!
3. Optional: Top with coconut whipped cream and pinch of cayenne, ancho chili powder or cinnamon and poke in a cinnamon stick.

WAYS YOU CAN ADAPT OR ENHANCE THIS RECIPE
- This is rich and creamy made with coconut milk, but you can try with any other creamy milk, such as Cashew Milk (p.148).
- Add 1-2 T. almond butter to mixture.

Orange JULIA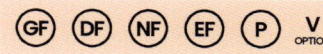

A healthy alternative to an Orange Julius. This is simple to make and tastes fresh.
I like it with very little sweetener, but you can adjust sweetener to your liking.

1 serving. *(Simply multiply by number of servings desired.)*

INGREDIENTS
½ cup freshly squeezed **orange juice**
½ cup **coconut milk** *(can of full fat or light)*
2 tsp. **honey**, or up to 2 T., to taste *(for V: use pure maple syrup or coconut nectar)*
½ tsp. **pure vanilla extract**
3 **ice cubes**

INSTRUCTIONS
1. Combine all ingredients in blender and blend on high until smooth and foamy. Start with just 2 tsp. of honey and slowly add more, if needed.
2. Pour into drinking glass and enjoy immediately.

Citrus MARTINI

My favorite martini. And somewhat healthy. Need I say more?!

INGREDIENTS
1 **fresh pink grapefruit**
2 large **fresh oranges**
2 **fresh limes**
1 large or 2 small **fresh lemons**
2 oz. **gin or vodka** *(mandarin or lemon vodka are nice)*
2 oz. **Cointreau** *(or other orange liqueur)*
2 oz. **Limoncello** or **ginger liqueur** *(...or just more Cointreau)*

INSTRUCTIONS
1. Make fresh juice from the grapefruit, oranges, limes and lemons. This should make close to 1½ cups of juice. Put this aside.
2. **For 3-4 martinis:** Mix all ingredients together with ice and strain/pour into martini glasses.
3. **For 1 martini:** Take ½ cup of the juice mixture and put it in a martini shaker with ice. Add ¾ oz. each of the 3 alcohols. Strain/pour into martini glass.
4. Store the remaining citrus juice in a sealed container for another martini the next day.)

WAYS YOU CAN ADAPT OR ENHANCE THIS RECIPE
- If you like a stronger martini, use less juice.
- Garnish ideas:
  - Rim each glass with a mixture of salt, sugar, and zest of any or all of the citrus (first dip ¼" of the rim in lemon or lime juice).
  - Add 3 frozen cranberries, blueberries, raspberries to each martini.
  - Add a half slice of orange, lemon or lime to the rim of each martini or thread wedges of lemon and lime onto skewer and place across top of martini glass.

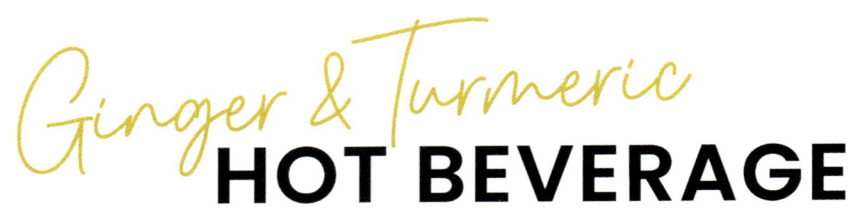
Ginger & Turmeric HOT BEVERAGE

GF | DF | NF | EF | P | V OPTION

This delicious and warming drink can be made in 5 minutes and contains anti-inflammatory properties (that help with brain and joint function, arthritis, bursitis and other musculoskeletal issues). It contains several healthy nutrients, including manganese, iron and vitamin K. When you want something warming and comforting, this hits the spot. It is recommended to drink daily because of the health benefits. This beverage calms the digestive system, so ideally drink it before bedtime. Be sure to check out the iced frappé version below.

Makes 2-3 servings

INGREDIENTS

2 T. **honey** *(for V: substitute with healthy sweetener of choice)*
1 packed tsp. freshly grated **ginger root**
1 tsp. **turmeric powder** *(or freshly grated turmeric)*
½ tsp. each of **ground ginger, cinnamon** & **cardamom** *(or more to taste)*
¼ tsp. **black pepper** *(see Tips)*
14-oz. can **coconut milk**, full fat or light *(see alternative milk options below)*
Hot water

INSTRUCTIONS

1. Place all ingredients in blender and blend until combined.
2. Pour into medium saucepan and heat through.
3. Add ¼ cup to 1 cup of hot water, depending on your taste.
4. Pour into mugs and serve with cinnamon stick or a sprinkle of cinnamon.
5. Store any remaining mixture in a sealed jar in fridge for up to 5 days.

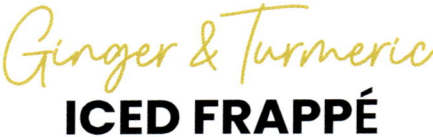
Ginger & Turmeric ICED FRAPPÉ

This is absolutely delicious! My new go-to summer beverage. Follow step #1 above, (omitting the added hot water) and then blend with plenty of ice. (Or pour over ice, if you prefer.)

TIPS
• Including black pepper with turmeric is important—it enhances absorption of turmeric's anti-inflammatory properties.

WAYS YOU CAN ADAPT OR ENHANCE THIS RECIPE
• Use alternate milk of choice. I've used coconut milk, homemade Cashew Milk (p.148) and Almond Milk (p.147). Try to avoid dairy milk—it can be inflammatory, which slightly defeats the purpose of an anti-inflammatory drink.
• You can add more freshly grated ginger and turmeric than the recipe calls for. This will give you more anti-inflammatory benefits. Note: Turmeric can be bitter, so be careful not to add too much.
• Add more or less sweetener, as desired.

SNACKS & "JUST FOR KIDS"

SNACKS

Caramel Corn with Macadamia Nuts *104*

Honey Butter Coconut Chips & 3-Seed Coconut Clusters *105*

Fudgsicles *107*

Candied Maple Walnuts and Candied Maple Pumpkin Seeds *108*

Orange Creamsicles *109*

Power Balls *109*

Apple Chips *110*

Vanilla & Lemon Custard Fruit Dip *113*

Salty, Sweet & Spicy Maple Pecans *114*

"JUST FOR KIDS"... of any age!

Just for Kids Recipes and Ideas *116-117*

Fruit on a Stick *119*

Mini Chocolate Cups with Various Fillings *120*

Banana Soft Serve Ice Cream *121*

Chocolate Chip Cookie Dough in Chocolate Cups *123*

Chocolate Popcorn *124*

Sprinkles *125*

Toasted Almonds 'n Honey Rice Crispy Squares *127*

Double Chocolate Fudge Mini Tarts *129*

CARAMEL CORN
with Macadamia Nuts

I admit, I have a weakness for Caramel Corn. Did you know popcorn contains vitamins, minerals, dietary fibre and polyphenol antioxidants? (Try to purchase organic popcorn to avoid GMO and chemicals.) I now can be guilt-free when I eat this healthy adaptation of traditional caramel corn. The macadamia nuts are a delicious addition; however, you can omit them, or substitute with other nuts (see below). This makes a great gift—fill a cellophane bag or sealed container and tie with a ribbon. Enjoy at Christmas, Halloween, Thanksgiving... or for family movie night. *Caution: Addictive!*

INGREDIENTS

10-12 cups **popped popcorn** *(⅓ cup kernels)*
3 cups **macadamia nuts** *(optional—see Adaptations below)*
½ cup **grass-fed butter** *(preferably unsalted)*
1 cup **coconut sugar**
¼ cup **honey** *(or coconut nectar)*
½ tsp. **sea salt** *(omit if using flaked salt later)*
½ tsp. **baking soda**
Optional: 2-3 pinches **flaked sea salt** for "salted caramel corn"

INSTRUCTIONS

1. Preheat the oven to 200° F.
2. Pop the ⅓ cup of popcorn and place into a large bowl. Remove unpopped kernels.
3. Spread nuts on top of the popped corn.
4. In a large saucepan, melt the butter; then stir in coconut sugar, honey and salt. Heat to boiling on high, stirring occasionally. Lower temperature to medium or low, but keep it at a low boil for 5 minutes, **without stirring**. Watch it doesn't boil over.
5. Remove from heat. Stir in baking soda until foamy.
6. Pour this over the popcorn & nuts and toss with 2 large spoons until popcorn is evenly coated (do this quickly!). **Be careful—it's very hot!**
7. Divide mixture onto 2 ungreased rimmed cookie sheets or baking pans.
8. Bake 1 hour, stirring every 15 minutes.
9. Once done, spread over parchment paper to cool. (If using flaked sea salt, sprinkle on at this point.) Cool completely, about 30 minutes.
10. Once cooled, if you have large chunks, break them down into more bite sized pieces. Store in sealed container.

WAYS YOU CAN ADAPT OR ENHANCE THIS RECIPE
• *For just "caramel corn", omit macadamia nuts. Or you can substitute macadamia nuts for raw or roasted nuts, such as pecans, almonds, walnuts, cashews or mixed nuts. If you use salted nuts, omit all salt in recipe.*
• *NF: Omit nuts or substitute with raw pumpkin, sunflower or sesame seeds.*
• *For a Chocolate and Caramel Corn Popcorn Duo, combine this recipe with Chocolate Popcorn (p.124).*
• *Try your own "Chicago Mix" by making a healthy cheese popcorn and combining it with this recipe.*

Honey Butter COCONUT CHIPS

GF | DF | NF | EF | V | P

For coconut lovers! I was just playing in the kitchen one day and came up with this recipe. Such a delicious snack! Healthy and easy to make! You can use this as a topping on Lemon Cashew Cheesecake (p.63), Blueberry Instant Ice Cream (p. 50), Banana Soft-Serve Ice Cream (p.121), or add to a Parfait (p.54).

INGREDIENTS

2½ cups **unsweetened coconut flakes** *(see Tips)*
1 T. plus 1 tsp. **homemade ghee** or **butter** *(for V: use coconut oil or vegan butter)*
2 T. **honey** *(for V: use coconut nectar)*
¾ tsp. **vanilla powder** *(or 1 tsp. pure vanilla extract)*
¼ tsp. **sea salt**, optional

INSTRUCTIONS

1. Place coconut chips in large bowl.
2. In a small saucepan over medium heat, melt ghee or coconut oil. When it is almost melted, add honey until honey is soft and pourable.
3. Remove from heat and add vanilla and whisk ingredients to blend well.
4. Pour warm mixture over coconut chips. Toss to coat.
5. Bake at 325° F about 8-10 minutes, until golden.
IMPORTANT NOTE: Check often to prevent burning. Toss, if necessary, to ensure even cooking.
6. Spread mixture out onto parchment to cool. (They will get crispier as they cool.) Let cool completely before storing in airtight container.

3-Seed COCONUT CLUSTERS

INGREDIENTS

1 T. **sesame seeds**
1 tsp. **chia seeds** *(or hemp seeds)*
1 tsp. **flax seeds**
1-2 T. **sliced almonds**
½ tsp. **ground ginger** *(optional)*

INSTRUCTIONS

• Same recipe and method as above, but stir in additional ingredients into the mixture in step #4 above.
• Form into clusters before baking.

TIPS
• Flaked coconut is sometimes called coconut chips or ribbons. Do not use shredded coconut.

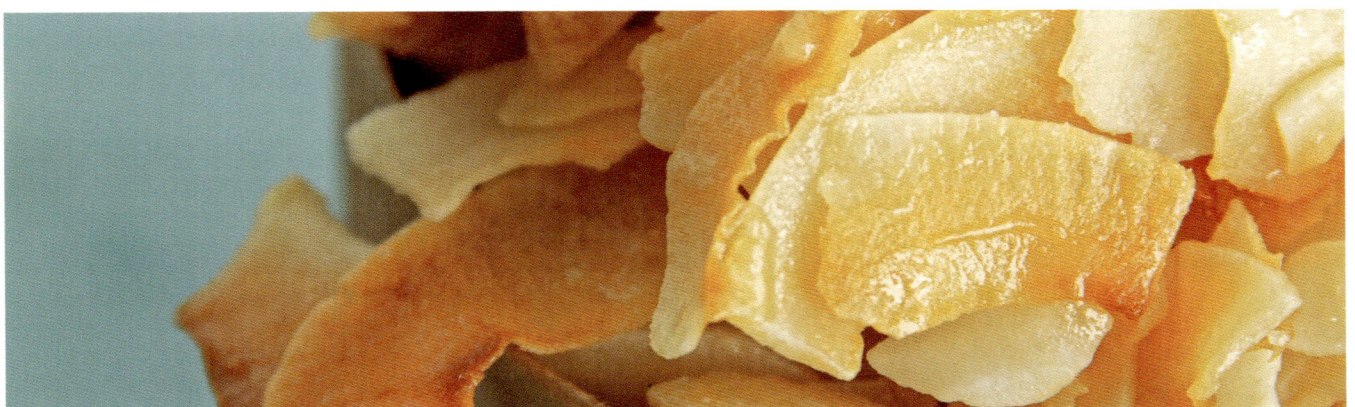

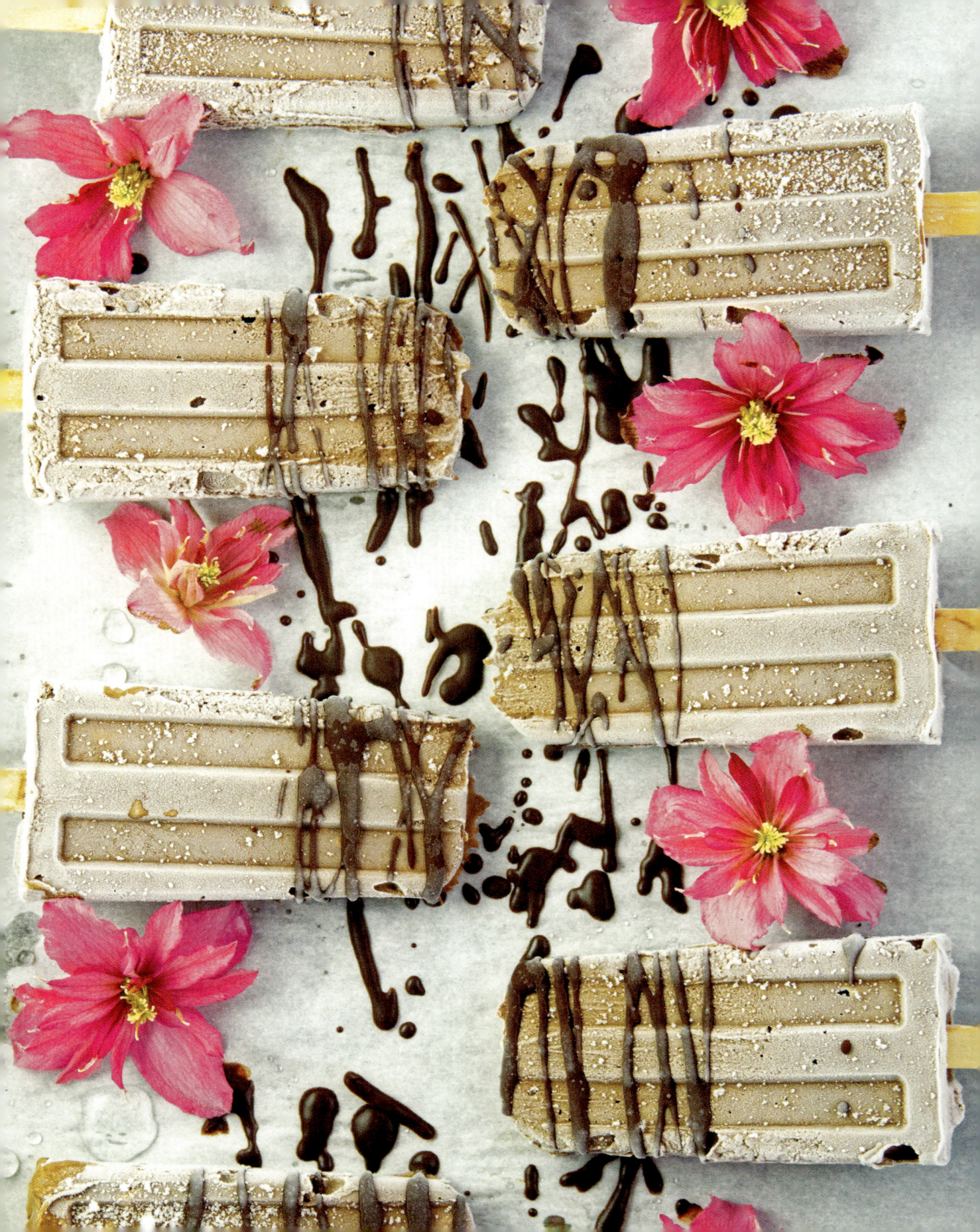

Fudgsicles

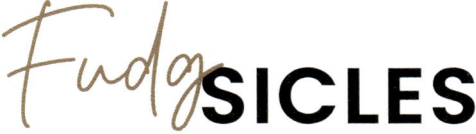

You won't believe how good these are—they taste amazingly like the real fudgsicle from days gone by! But thankfully they are made without the dairy, refined sugar and other additives that are in the commercial ones. This was a happy "accident"—I created them from leftover OMG Chocolate Avocado Pudding (p.85). The avocado is what makes them so creamy, yet you don't taste the avocado. They are so easy to make—just throw all ingredients in a blender and pour into molds and freeze. These are definitely for the kid in all of us!
Be sure to also check out the Fudgsicle's nostalgic cousin, the Orange Creamsicle (p.109)!

Makes approximately 12-14, depending on size of molds

INGREDIENTS

2 large *(or 3 small)* **ripe avocados**
½ cup **dates**, pits removed and chopped *(soaked in ½ cup hot water for 20 minutes...keep and use water!)*
½ cup **pure maple syrup** *(or more, to taste)*
⅓ cup **cacao powder** *(use up to ¾ cup for more intense chocolate flavour)*
14-oz. can **full-fat coconut milk**
1 tsp. **pure vanilla extract**
pinch **sea salt**

You will need fudgsicle/popsicle mold and popsicle sticks! *(If you don't have a mold, see Tips.)*

INSTRUCTIONS

1. Place all ingredients in a food processor or high-speed blender (including saved water). Blend until smooth. Taste. Add more cacao powder or maple syrup, if desired.
2. Pour into molds, insert sticks and freeze. (If you don't have a mold, *see Tips*.)

TIPS
- I highly recommend getting a fudgsicle or popsicle mold; however, if you don't have one, you can use Dixie cups— just fill, cover each with tin foil, and make a small slit in top to insert stick before freezing.

WAYS YOU CAN ADAPT OR ENHANCE THIS RECIPE
- I like to poke in 1 or 2 slices of strawberry or banana into each fudgsicle before freezing. Try adding other fruit.
- Stir in 1-2 tsp. of dark chocolate chunks, chocolate chips, or cacao nibs.
- Drizzle with chocolate sauce immediately after they come out of the freezer molds with a simple homemade Chocolate Sauce (p.135).
- Add one of the following to the mixture in the blender: ½ tsp. mint extract for "chocolate mint fudgsicles", or ½ cup peanut butter for the chocolate peanut butter cup flavour. Or for "cappuccino" fudgsicle, mix in 1 T. (or more, to taste) finely ground coffee, 1-2 tsp. instant espresso, or 1-2 oz. strong brewed espresso.
- Boozy version: Add 2-3 T. of your favorite liquor or liqueur, such as Grand Marnier, Kahlua, Sambuca, Cinnamon Whiskey, Amaretto, etc. (Or add 1 tsp. to each fudgsicle.)
- For Entertaining: Guests can dip their Fudgsicle in small bowls of room temperature (or slightly heated) Spiced Caramel Sauce (p.132) or Chocolate Chili Ganache (p.136). Then dip fudgsicle in another small bowl of roasted and finely chopped hazelnuts. Yum!!

Candied MAPLE WALNUTS

GF DF EF V P

Oh, so Canadian!
This is a great healthy snack! And somewhat addictive! Try them sprinkled on top of Pumpkin Spice Custard Cups (p. 58) or on top of a Parfait (p. 54). They are also excellent sprinkled on a tossed green salad with crumbled goat cheese and sliced pears. Or for an appetizer, brie baked with sprigs of thyme or rosemary, then drizzled with balsamic reduction and topped with candied maple walnuts before serving.

INGREDIENTS

1½ cups **raw walnut halves** *(or large pieces)*

¼ cup **pure maple syrup** *(can add 1-2 T. more if prefer sweeter)*

Optional: ¼-½ tsp. **coarse sea salt** *(or fleur de sel or Maldon sea salt flakes)*

WAYS YOU CAN ADAPT OR ENHANCE THIS RECIPE

• *Delicious made with other nuts or seeds: pecans, almonds, hazelnuts, pistachios, macadamias, sesame seeds and sunflower seeds.*

INSTRUCTIONS

1. Place walnuts in small skillet on medium heat. Dry roast for 3-5 minutes, stirring often, being careful not to burn.
2. Add maple syrup to pan and stir continuously until liquid reduces and walnuts appear to have soaked up most of the maple syrup, about 4 minutes (depending on your skillet and heat source).
3. Carefully spoon mixture onto parchment paper. (**Be careful**...it's very hot and can burn your skin.)
4. Sprinkle with sea salt, if using.
5. Let cool at room temperature or in fridge.
6. Store in airtight container in fridge.

Candied MAPLE PUMPKIN SEEDS

Same recipe as above, but replace walnuts with **1¼ cups raw pumpkin seeds.**

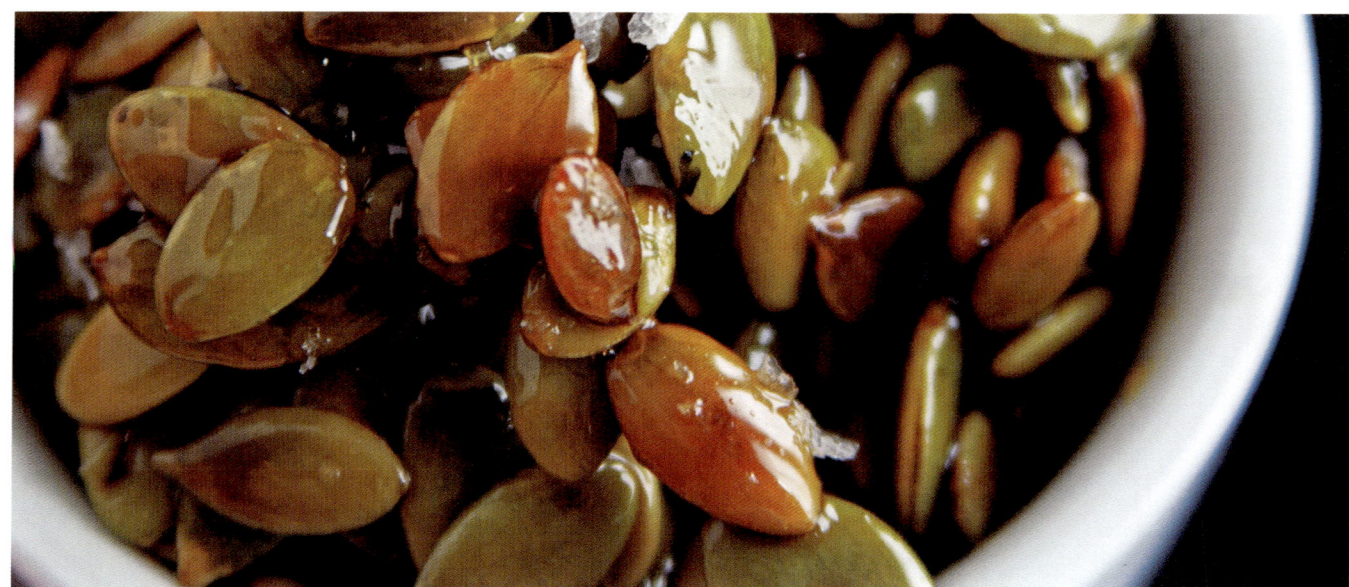

Orange CREAMSICLES

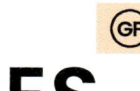

Yes…these taste like the original frozen treats of summers gone by…minus the refined sugar, dairy, and questionable ingredients. I was playing with the Lemon & Lime Frozen Mini Cheesecakes (p. 57) using fresh orange juice. Then I added some ingredients from the Orange Julia (p.101) recipe and…Voila!…Creamsicles! These babies are made with coconut milk, raw cashews and honey, so are filled with protein, vitamin C, magnesium, potassium, iron and dietary fibre.

Makes about 5, depending on size of popsicle mold

INGREDIENTS

½ cup **raw cashews**, soaked in water for minimum 2 hours or overnight in fridge
½ cup of **full-fat coconut milk**
¼ cup **mild-tasting honey** *(for V: use coconut nectar or pure maple syrup)*
2 **oranges**, zested then juiced *(juice to measure ½ cup)*
1 tsp. **pure vanilla extract**
Optional: ¼ tsp. **orange extract** *(or 1 or 2 drops of food grade orange essential oil)*
Popsicle or fudgsicle mold and popsicle sticks *(see Tips)*

INSTRUCTIONS

1. Rinse and drain cashews.
2. Place all ingredients into a high-speed blender and puree until mixture is smooth and creamy.
3. Pour mixture into fudgsicle or popsicle molds, insert sticks and freeze.

TIPS

• I highly recommend getting a fudgsicle or popsicle mold; however, if you don't have one, you can use Dixie cups—just fill, cover each with tin foil, and make a small slit in top to insert stick before freezing.

WAYS YOU CAN ADAPT OR ENHANCE THIS RECIPE

• *To make Orange Creamsicle Frozen Mini Cheesecakes:* Use the "crust" from Lemon & Lime Frozen Mini Cheesecakes (p.57) or Brown Butter & Rosemary Chocolate Tartlets (p.71). Press the crust mixture firmly into the bottom of 18-24 mini muffin cups or 6-8 regular-sized muffin cups (lined with paper liners). Pour Orange Creamsicles mixture on top. Freeze for 2-4 hours. Enjoy frozen!

Power BALLS

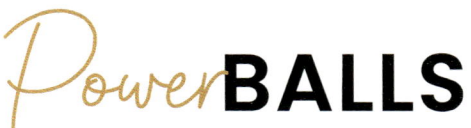 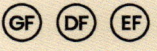

This is a one-bowl, no bake, fast recipe. A great snack for work, school, the car, or for hiking and activities. This is a very flexible recipe—you can change and alter ingredients as you wish (see below), as long as you create a mixture that holds together when pressed into a ball shape. My favorite additions are hemp seeds and chocolate chips or dried cranberries. The key word here is "power"—these are filled with protein, fibre, iron, potassium and calcium.

Makes 24 balls

INGREDIENTS

1¼ cups **rolled oats**
1 cup **peanut butter** *(or nut or seed butter of choice)*
⅓ cup **honey** *(for V: use coconut nectar or pure maple syrup)*
¼ cup **sesame seeds**
½ cup **unsweetened shredded coconut** *(plus extra to roll balls in)*

INSTRUCTIONS

1. Mix ingredients in large bowl.
2. Make into balls and roll to coat in extra coconut (or hemp seeds).
3. Store in sealed container.

WAYS YOU CAN ADAPT OR ENHANCE THIS RECIPE

• *Substitute rolled oats with other "flakes" (i.e. rye, barley, quinoa, kamut, etc.).*
• *Optional Additions: For added protein, add 2-3 T. hemp seeds to mixture and roll balls in hemp seeds. Add small amount of chocolate chips, chopped, dried fruit such as cranberries, mango, dates or apricots, any nuts or seeds (peanuts, sunflower seeds, chia seeds, pumpkin seeds, pecans, walnuts, brazil nuts, etc.).*

Apple CHIPS

Homemade apple chips are a delicious and healthy snack. Just one ingredient—apples! Nothing is added; only moisture is removed. Make big batches of these and store them in a tightly sealed container; they'll store for months. I use a coring tool and a mandolin (slicing machine), and a 9-tray dehydrator to make these. I have also offered an oven method. You can also use an air fryer—just follow air fryer instructions. You've got to love nature's own candy.

INGREDIENTS: Apples *(Jona Gold and Gala are my favorite, but you can use any kind)*

DEHYDRATOR METHOD (RECOMMENDED)

1. Wash, dry and core apples. (Leave skin on to keep good fibre, vitamins and minerals.)
2. Slice apples very thinly and evenly, preferably using a mandolin slicer. (I use the 1.5mm thickness setting.)
3. I don't mind my apples turning a golden color—a natural oxidation process. (If you like, however, you can dip slices in anti-browning solution of ¼ cup lemon juice in 1 quart of water. Remove slices and pat dry.)
4. Place apple slices in a single layer on dehydrator racks and dehydrate at 115° F for 3-12 hours (depending on type of apples, humidity, thickness of slices, and how dry you like them—I like mine best at the 4-5 hour point).
5. After 4 hours, check for any moisture on outside and inside—rip a slice in half to see if there is any moisture on the inside. If there is any moisture, dehydrate longer. (Dehydrate as long as you like—they will eventually dry to a crispier texture and, if dehydrated enough, will crispen more when they cool. I like them when they are still soft and chewy, but some people like them crispy.)
6. Allow to cool completely before storing in an airtight container or Ziploc bag. Store in a dry, cool, dark place for several months.

CONVECTION OVEN METHOD

1. Follow the steps beside, but instead use a convection oven set at the lowest "convection bake" temperature, about 150° F (65°C). If oven does not set under 200° F, then prop door open slightly to allow for air circulation and moisture to escape from the oven. (You don't want to bake the apples—you just want to remove the moisture with circulating warm air.)
2. Arrange apple slices on wire baking or cooling racks and position in oven.
3. Dehydrate 3-12 hours. Times vary due to humidity levels, ovens, temperature, apple varieties, thickness of apples, and how soft or dry you like them. Just keep checking every hour after the 3-hour point.

TIPS
• *If you keep the dehydrating temperature under 118° F, some of the enzymes and nutrients will not be lost. This aligns with the philosophy of "raw food" cooking and baking.*

WAYS YOU CAN ADAPT OR ENHANCE THIS RECIPE
• *Sprinkle apple chips with a little cinnamon before dehydrating.*
• *I like to eat apple chips as they are, but for a special treat, dip half of the dried apple chips in Chocolate Sauce (135-136), Caramel Sauce (p.131-133), Vanilla & Lemon Custard Fruit Dip (p.113), Lemon Curd made with Honey (p.145), Blueberry Sauce (p.142), Pecan Praline Butter (p.143), Raspberry or Mango Coulis (p.142), or any nut butter.*

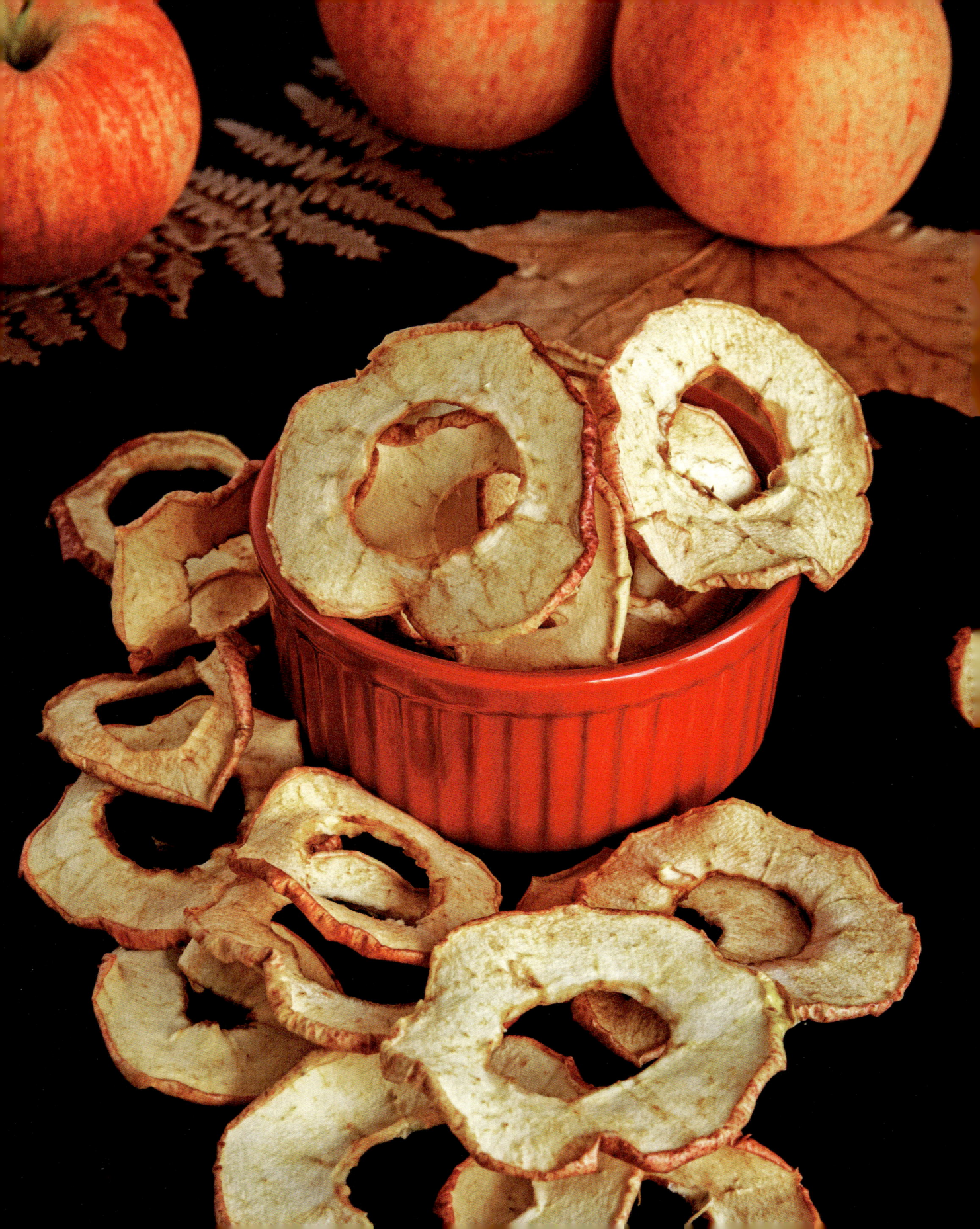

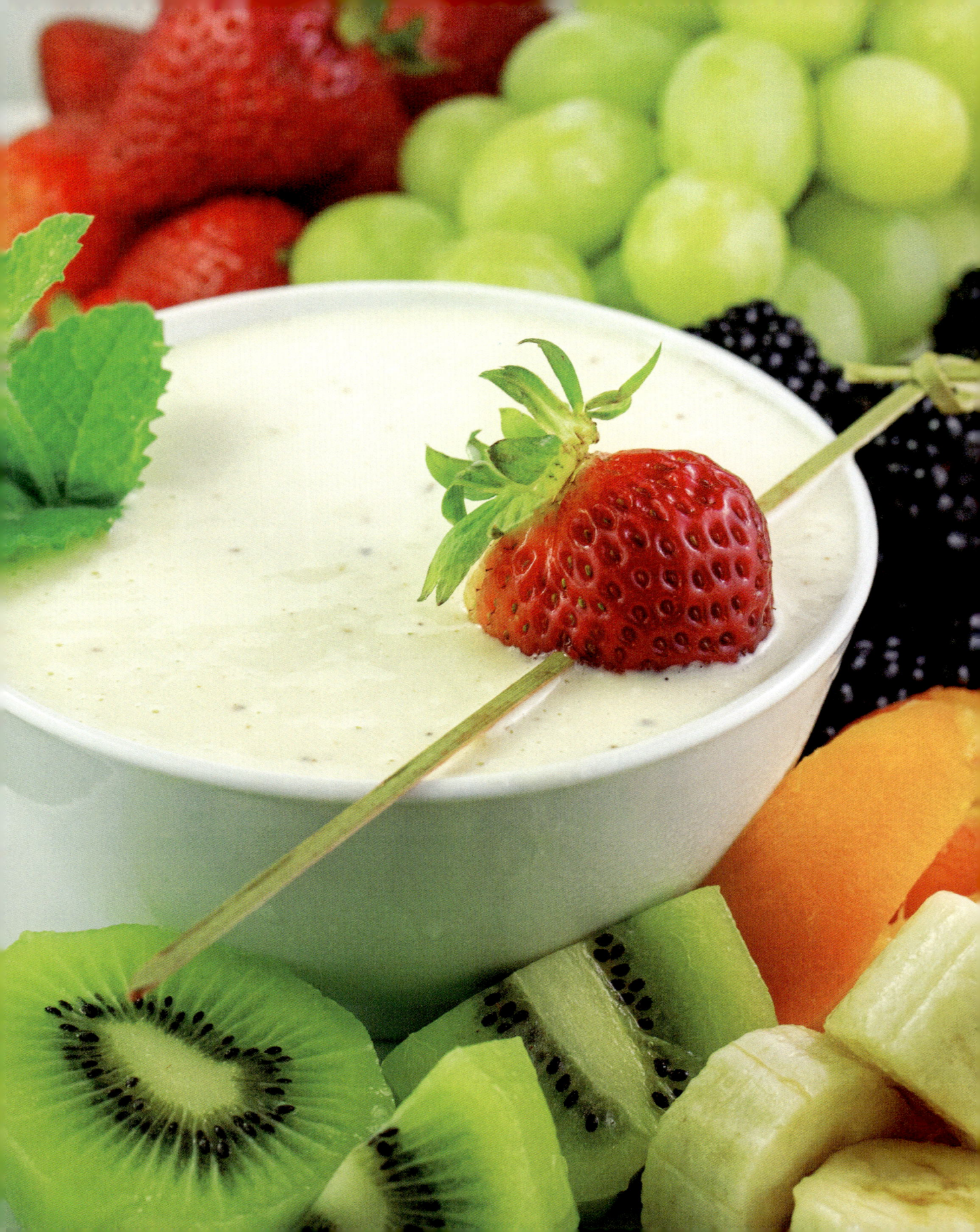

Vanilla & Lemon
CUSTARD FRUIT DIP

I love, love, love this dip. I can't get enough of it. I love the custard flavour. And it always surprises me how much I love the combination of vanilla, lemon and nutmeg flavours. I end up eating a lot of fruit because I like the dip so much. This is a smart and healthy way to get your children and family to eat more fruit, too! My favourite fruits to dip are banana, strawberry, plum and watermelon…although any fresh fruit is good! I haven't met a fruit that doesn't like this dip. I do warn you, however…you may not ever want to eat fresh fruit on its own again.

Makes about 3 cups

INGREDIENTS

½ cup **honey**
14-oz. can **full-fat coconut milk**
6 large **egg yolks**
1 T. **organic cornstarch** *(for P: use arrowroot starch)*
1 tsp. **unflavoured gelatin**
2 T. **grass-fed butter** *(for DF: use vegan butter)*
4 tsp. **freshly squeezed lemon juice** *(or ¼ tsp. lemon extract)*
4 tsp. **pure vanilla extract** *(see Adaptations below for other vanilla options)*
½ tsp. **nutmeg** *(preferably freshly grated)*

INSTRUCTIONS

1. Sprinkle the gelatin over 2 tsp. water and let sit to bloom for 10 minutes.
2. In medium or large saucepan, heat honey. Then add coconut milk. Heat and let simmer 4 minutes. Do not boil, but mixture should be steaming hot.
3. In a medium or large bowl, whisk egg yolks and cornstarch until frothy and light colour, about 2 minutes.
4. Gradually pour hot honey-coconut milk mixture into eggs, whisking continuously. (Adding very gradually is important so eggs don't curdle.)
5. Pour all the mixture back into the saucepan on medium heat, stirring **continuously** with a silicone spatula until mixture is thick and bubbly.
6. Remove from heat. Immediately add bloomed gelatin and butter. Whisk for about 1 minute. Pour mixture into a small bowl and let mixture sit for 5 minutes. (If there are any lumps, push the mixture through a fine sieve into the bowl.)
7. Whisk in lemon juice, vanilla extract and nutmeg.
8. Let cool another 5 minutes and then cover with plastic wrap (or a circle of parchment paper), pushing the plastic down to touch surface of custard. Chill in fridge 3 hours or overnight. Store in sealed container in fridge for up one week.

TIPS
- *Get a good quality, organic, full-fat coconut milk. I like Whole Foods 365 the best—it contains a good amount of coconut cream and the texture is smooth. Also good are Native Forest and Thai brands.*
- ***Any fresh fruit makes for good dippables! Some ideas are:** Bananas, strawberries, grapes, kiwifruit, blueberries, raspberries, blackberries, orange or grapefruit segments, peaches, nectarines, plums, figs, pineapple, mango, papaya, cantaloupe, honeydew melon, apples, cherries, pears, watermelon, star fruit, passion fruit.*
- *Check honey resource on p. 12 for delicious, mild-tasting, creamy raw honey. It's 100% pure Canadian, well-priced, and they deliver.*
- *See "Fruit on a Stick" (p.119) for more ideas.*

WAYS YOU CAN ADAPT OR ENHANCE THIS RECIPE
- *For a stronger vanilla flavour, omit vanilla extract and instead add seeds scraped from one vanilla pod (or use 1 tsp. vanilla powder) and add to honey/coconut milk mixture in step #2.*

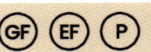
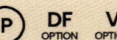

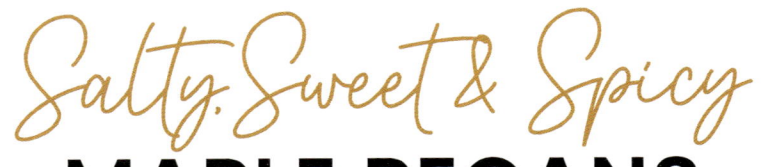

MAPLE PECANS

Everyone loves this snack! It's sweet, salty, spicy and crunchy... 4 of my favourite qualities in a snack. This is a Christmas time favourite of ours...and it makes a great gift, too. These are Dom's fave, and my friend Karen calls these "Patti's Perky Pecans".

Makes 4 cups

INGREDIENTS

1 lb. *(454 g)* **pecan halves** *(about 4 cups)*
1 T. **grass-fed butter** *(for V: use coconut oil)*
⅔ cup **pure maple syrup**
3 T. **maple sugar**
2 tsp. each of **ground cumin, sweet paprika, chili powder**
⅛ tsp. **cayenne** *(double if you like spicy)*
1 tsp. **sea salt**

INSTRUCTIONS

1. Position a rack in the center of the oven and preheat to 350° F.
2. Spread the pecans in a large cookie sheet or roasting pan and bake until lightly toasted, about 8 minutes.
3. Add butter to the same pan and stir to coat bottom of pan.
4. Pour maple syrup over the nuts and toss to coat well. Bake, stirring occasionally, until the nuts have absorbed most of the syrup, 10-15 minutes.
5. Mix the sugar and spices in a small bowl. Pour the nuts into a large bowl. Toss with a spoon, gradually adding the sugar mixture, until the nuts are coated with the sugar mixture.
6. Cool slightly and break apart any nuts that are sticking together. Pour onto a waxed paper sheet and cool completely.
7. They can be stored in an airtight container at room temperature for up to 1 week

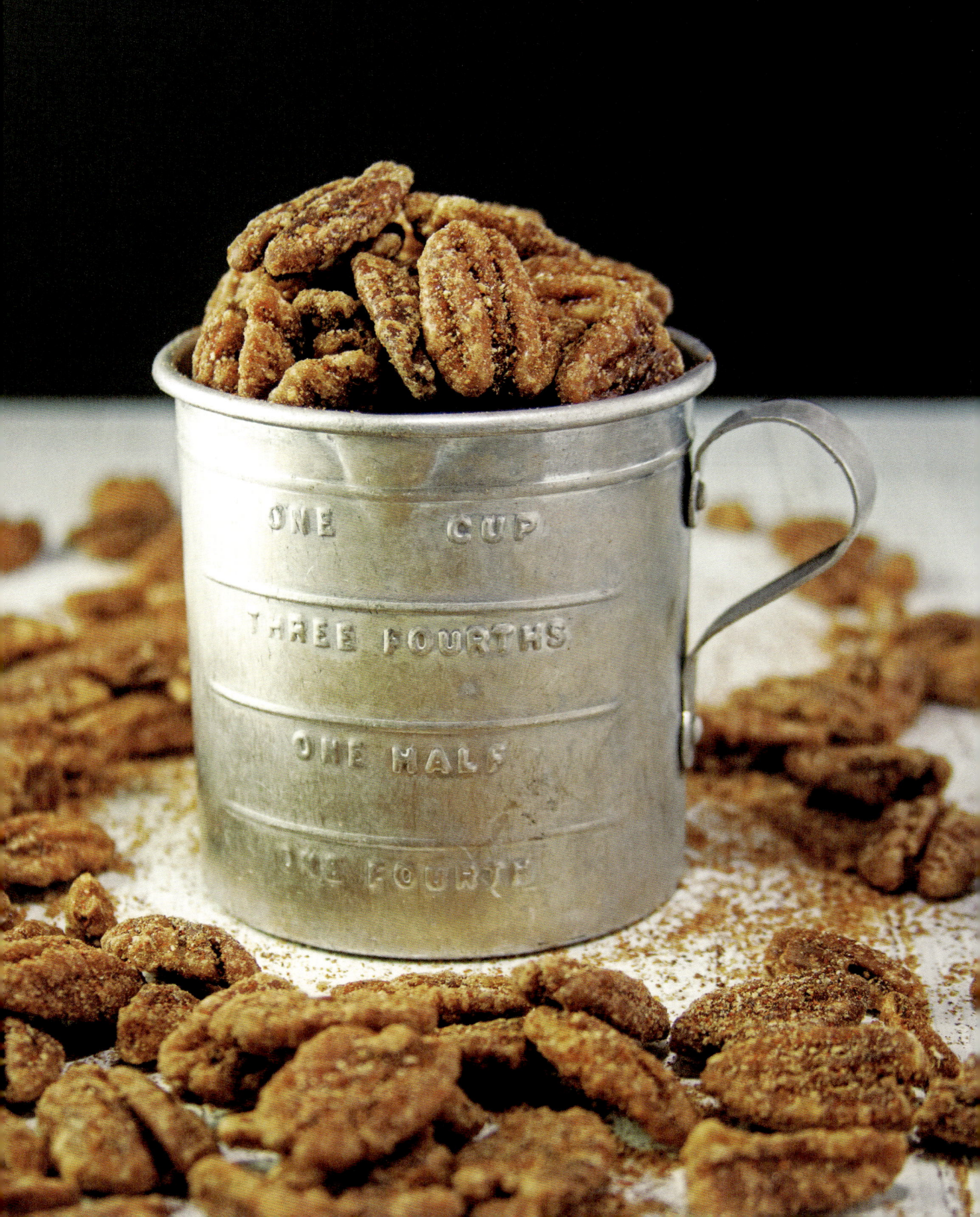

"JUST FOR KIDS"
OF ANY AGE

Kids love to bake and they love sweets. Why not get them interested at a young age in delicious, healthy choices that will develop a healthy sweet tooth and a healthy attitude towards food. Baking can be so much fun! But be sure kids get adult help with these. Safety comes first! There is one rule in this section: Kids get to lick the bowl!

Here are some recipes and recipe ideas that you can make with kids:

- **Banana Ice cream** - Several flavour variations and additions (see p.121).
- **Popsicles** - Make with fruit blended with water, yogurt or coconut milk.
- **Fudgsicles** - (p.107)
- **Fruit and Dips** - (p.119 & 113)
- **Apple & PB** - Cut apple into wedges arranged in circle in a bowl. Serve with small amount of peanut butter in the centre.
- **Apple Donuts** - Cut ¼" slices of apple. Then cut out holes in the middle into shapes (use cookie cutters). Fill with peanut butter, almond butter, No-Cook Fruit Jam (p.146), or Caramel Sauce (p.131-133) and sandwich with another apple slice that has no hole (like linzer cookies).
- **Pecan Rice Crispy Triangles** - (p.39)
- **Toasted Almonds 'n Honey Rice Crispy Squares** - (p.127)
- **Apple Chips** - (p.110) Eat as is or dip in any Chocolate Sauce (p.135-136) or Caramel Sauce (p.131-133) and then sprinkle with hemp seeds or Sprinkles (p.125).
- **Sprinkles** - Make your own (p.125).
- **Power Balls** - (p.109) Make ingredient changes just for fun.
- **Frozen Yogurt Blueberries** – Thread a few fresh or frozen blueberries onto a skewer or toothpick, then dip in Greek Yogurt. Freeze. Eat frozen. (Or spoon yogurt into mini muffin cups with berries poked in. Sprinkle granola on top of each, then freeze.)
- **Frozen Yogurt Bark** - Spread unsweetened Greek yogurt onto a lined baking sheet. Sprinkle various toppings on, such as nuts, granola, dried or fresh fruit, chocolate chips, Sprinkles (p.125). Freeze until firm. Break into pieces and eat immediately.
- **Fruit Lollies** - Thread large banana chunks, pineapple chunks, apple slices, orange segments (or any fruit piece) onto lollipop or popsicle sticks, or skewers. Roll in warmed Chocolate Sauce (p.135), warmed Caramel Sauce (p.131-133), or Raspberry Coulis (p.142) and then dip in bowls of various items such as crispy rice cereal, shredded coconut, hemp seeds, chopped nuts, seeds, sea salt, goji berries, dried blueberries, or Sprinkles (p.125). Freeze. Eat frozen.
- **Chocolate Circles** (French Mendiants) - Adults make the small chocolate circles (see p.75). Kids add toppings, such as chopped nuts, sliced dried apricots, coconut flakes, etc. Place in fridge for 5 or 10 minutes to set.
- **Smoothies** - Make your own smoothies in a blender with fresh or frozen fruit and plain Greek yogurt, Cashew Cream (p.148), or plant-based milk. Be creative!
- **Trail Mix** - Mix together assorted nuts, seeds and chocolate chips.
- **Frozen Grapes** - Simply freeze washed, fresh grapes. Eat frozen. Or use as "ice cubes" in a beverage.
- **Fruit Leather** (fruit roll-ups) - Blend any juicy fruit in blender, such as berries, peaches, kiwi or mango and pour onto dehydrator sheets and spread thinly and evenly. Dehydrate at 115 F. until consistency of fruit leather.
- **Dried Fruit & Chocolate Dips** - Take Apple Chips (p.110) or pieces of dried fruit such as mango or apricots, and dip half in melted chocolate chips or warmed Chocolate Sauce (p.135-136). Then sprinkle with coconut, seeds, Sprinkles (p.125), chopped nuts or crispy rice cereal.

- **Apple Bites** - Spoon apple sauce into lined mini muffin cups or ice cube trays. (Optional: Place a small stick in each.) Freeze. Eat partially frozen.
- **Date Pops** - Put a medjool date on a toothpick or popsicle stick and dip in warmed Chocolate Sauce (p.135), warmed Caramel Sauce (p.131-133), or yogurt. Or stuff with nut butter and dip ½ in chocolate sauce. Or eat dates plain (like candy!).
- **Raw Fruit Pizza** - Make raw crust for Berrylicious Cheesecake (p.49) and press onto 8" round, flat pan. Spread on Vanilla & Lemon Custard Fruit Dip (p.113) and top with any fresh fruit...ie. orange segments, kiwi slices, sliced bananas, berries, etc. Place fruit in a circular pattern starting at outside and working inwards. Brush with honey-sweetened lemon juice or warmed peach or apricot jam. Refrigerate until set. Cut like a pizza.
- **Layered Parfait** - (p.54) Have fun making up different layers.
- **Chocolate Almond Milk** - Make Almond Milk (p.147), add melted chocolate chips, or Chocolate Sauce of choice (p.135-136). Whisk or blend.
- **Mexican Hot Chocolate** - (p.100) Forego the chili powder and cayenne.
- **Dessert Jars**: Fill small mason jars with layers of broken cookies, Chia Jam (p.146), diced fresh fruit, and Fruit Dip (p.119 & 113) or yogurt. Use many recipes from this book, such as OMG! Chocolate Avocado Pudding (p.85), layered with bananas and Granola (p.95). Make up your own creations!
- **Cookie Sandwiches** - Take any two cookies and fill with chilled Hazel-Nut-Ella Chocolate Spread (p.144), Caramel Sauce (p.131-133) or Date Paste (p.143). Or fill with ice cream and freeze.
- **Caramel Corn** - (p.104) Adult makes this—Kids eat it! Caution: Hot mixture can burn.
- **Chocolate Chip Cookie Dough in Chocolate Cups** - (p.123) Adults guide chocolate cup making.
- **Mini Chocolate Cups with Fillings** - (p.120) Adults guide chocolate cup making. Kids fill cups with various filling ideas provided.
- **Chocolate Brownies** - (p.77) Make without espresso. Cool, and top with Sugarless Chocolate Frosting (p.136). Slice into squares and top each with dollop of coconut whipped cream and sprinkle of cacao nibs, or a drizzle of Caramel Sauce (p.131-133).
- **Chocolate Fondue** - Make choice of Chocolate Sauce (p.135) and bring to warm temperature (adults assist). Dip various pieces of fresh fruit, dried fruit, pieces of muffins or cake into sauce. Optional: Then dip into toppings — fill small bowls with unsweetened shredded coconut, cacao nibs, chopped nuts, seeds, crispy rice cereal, Sprinkles (p.125), etc. A fun family affair!
- **Thumbprint Cookies** - Make Banana Oatmeal Sugar-Free Cookies (p.29) and fill with No-Cook Fruit Jam (p.146), or with a few chocolate chips. Or make an indentation before baking and leave empty for baking, then once cookies are baked and cooled, fill with peanut butter mixed with chocolate chips, Honey Butter Coconut Chips (p.105), Candied Maple Walnuts or Pumpkin Seeds (p.108), a fresh strawberry (or other fruit) drizzled with warmed honey or melted chocolate, or whatever kids can come up with.
- **Triple Berry (Berrylicious) Cashew Cheesecake** - Adults guide the process but kids poke the frozen raspberries and blueberries into the filling.
- **Caramel Apple Wedges** - Think Caramel Apple but instead insert small skewer or popsicle sticks into wedges of Granny Smith apples and then dip into warmed Caramel Sauce (p.131-133). (If entertaining, keep caramel sauce warm in a small crockpot or fondue pot.) Consider topping with drizzle of warmed Chocolate Sauce (p.135. Or top with sea salt, cacao nibs, chocolate chips, chopped roasted nuts, hemp seeds, Sprinkles (p.125), or flaked coconut.
- **Caramel Apples** - Poke sticks into whole Granny Smith apples and then dip in warmed Caramel Sauce of your choice (p.131-133). Consider then dipping top half into chopped, roasted nuts or crispy rice cereal. Go all out with a drizzle of Chocolate Sauce (p.135) on top of that! Place on parchment-lined pan and chill in fridge to set.
- **Crunchy Chocolate Bites** - (p.91) These are easy-to-make mini chocolate bars. Try different fillings, flavours and toppings.
- **Dark Chocolate Pecan Clusters** - (p.87) Try variations or nut & fruit combination.
- **OMG! Chocolate Avocado Puddings** - (p.85) Have fun trying flavour and topping variations.

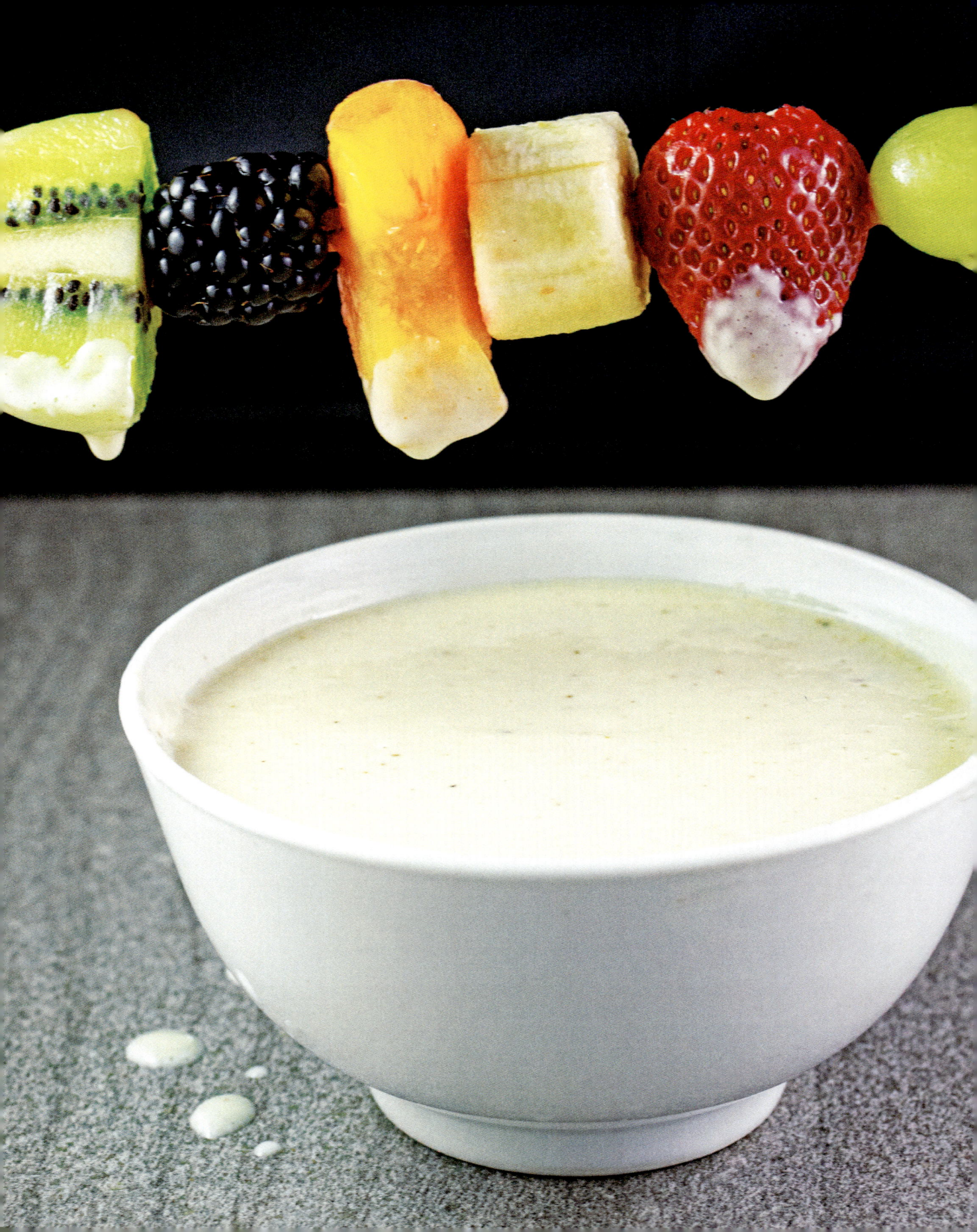

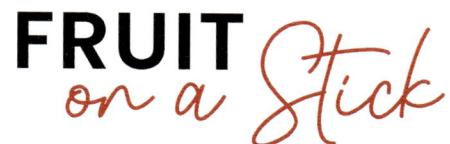

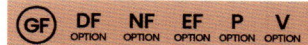

Dip pieces of fruit into various dips for a delicious and healthy snack. You can insert a bamboo skewer, popsicle stick or appetizer stick into each piece of fruit and lay them on a platter. Or insert the fruit-filled sticks into styrofoam and display vertically. After dipping the fruit in a sauce, perhaps drizzle with a caramel, chocolate or blueberry sauce and then sprinkle with your choice of topping. Think "Caramel Apple" by dipping apple wedges in caramel sauce! Caramel or chocolate sauces can be heated slowly or kept warm in a small crockpot or fondue pot for entertaining. (Safety alert—adults need to supervise.) Or keep it as simple as dipping apple wedges in almond butter, banana chunks in caramel sauce, or strawberries in chocolate sauce.

FRUIT
- apple wedges
- banana chunks
- strawberries
- pineapple chunks
- pear wedges
- mango chunks
- melon balls
- papaya chunks
- peach or nectarine wedges
- apricot halves
- cherries *(keep stem on and omit skewer)*
- grapes *(put 2 or 3 on one skewer)*
- orange segments
- starfruit "stars"
- kiwi halves
- plum halves
- watermelon chunks

DIPS
- Vanilla & Lemon Custard Fruit Dip (p.113)
- Caramel Sauce of choice (p.131-133)
- Chocolate Sauce of choice (p.135-136)
- Blueberry Sauce (p.142)
- Raspberry Coulis (p.142)
- Lemon Curd (p.145)
- Strawberry Cashew Cream (p.148)
- Coconut Chia Pudding *(just the pudding part)* (p.61)
- nut butter of choice *(or seed butter)*
- apple sauce
- coconut manna *(coconut butter)*, warmed/melted *(Caution: Let cool a little)*
- blackstrap molasses
- Greek yogurt
- pure maple syrup
- warmed honey or coconut nectar

TOPPINGS
- drizzle with another sauce *(think warmed caramel or chocolate sauce)*
- sprinkles or unsweetened shredded coconut
- chopped nuts
- hemp seeds
- cacao nibs *(or chocolate chips or shavings)*
- coconut
- coconut whipped cream

TIPS
- *To keep fruit such as apples and bananas from turning brown (oxidizing), simply brush a small amount of lemon juice over the pieces right after cutting.*

WAYS YOU CAN ADAPT OR ENHANCE THIS RECIPE
- *For a little variety and added protein and calcium, add cubes of semi-hard cheese to the skewers, such as cheddar.*

Mini CHOCOLATE CUPS
WITH VARIOUS FILLINGS

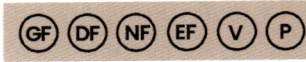

Get out your little paint brushes! These are easy to make, look decorative when filled, and filling ideas are endless. Kids—be creative and have fun coming up with filling ingredients!

Makes 12 mini cups *(Use silicone mini muffin cup liners. If using paper liners, be sure to get parchment or non-stick ones.)*

INGREDIENTS

⅔ cup *(100g or 3.7 oz)* **dark chocolate chips** *(bittersweet, 70-85% cacao) (I use Camino, organic bittersweet chocolate chips.) (See Adaptation below for refined sugar-free chocolate version.)*

INSTRUCTIONS

1. Melt chocolate slowly in bain marie (in a bowl over simmering water—don't let bowl touch water). (Temper chocolate, if you choose. Tempering instructions easily found online.) Remove from heat and let cool for 10 minutes.
2. Brush melted chocolate onto sides and bottom of silicone mini muffin cups, brushing up the sides as much as possible. If you have extra melted chocolate, give the sides an extra coat.
3. Place in fridge to set until ready to fill.
4. Spoon or pipe fillings into cups.

FILLING IDEAS

- OMG! Chocolate Avocado Pudding (p.85)
- Chocolate Chip Cookie Dough (p.123)
- Hazelnut-Ella Chocolate Spread (p.144)
- Candied Maple Walnuts (p.108)
- Salty, Sweet & Spicy Maple Pecans (p.114)
- Caramel Popcorn (p.104) or Chocolate Popcorn (p.124)
- Honey Butter Coconut Chips (p.105)
- Power Balls (p.109)
- Vanilla & Lemon Custard Fruit Dip (p.113)
- Strawberry Cashew Cream or Sweetened Thick Cashew Cream (p.148) topped with Sprinkles (p.125)
- Lemon Curd (p.145) or Vanilla & Lemon Custard Fruit Dip (p.113)
- Choice of Caramel Sauce (p.131-133) (chilled)
- Chocolate-Chili Ganache (p.136) or Sugarless Chocolate Frosting (p.136)
- Date Paste (p.143) or No-Cook Fruit Jam (p.146)
- Chocolate Espresso Pâté (p.82)
- Fresh fruit such as berries or chopped bananas
- Balsamic-roasted strawberries

TOPPINGS

Your favourite pudding, snacks, cereal, candies... or whatever you like!

- Top any of the above with a small dollop of coconut whipped cream, then a drizzle of Raspberry Coulis (p.142), Caramel Sauce (p.131-133) or Chocolate Sauce (p.135), then top with a whole raspberry, a slice of strawberry... or a pinch of cacao nibs or chocolate chips, crispy rice cereal, broken cookies, Sprinkles (p.125) or an edible flower.
- Adults only! – Fill with your favourite liqueur or shooter

WAYS YOU CAN ADAPT OR ENHANCE THIS RECIPE

- For refined sugar-free chocolate cups, use unsweetened chocolate. (I used Camino, organic unsweetened chocolate chips.) When melted, remove from heat and whisk in 1-2 T. pure maple syrup, coconut nectar or honey.

Banana SOFT SERVE ICE CREAM

(GF) (DF) (NF) (EF) (V) (P)

One Ingredient – Just Bananas! Don't be fooled by the simplicity of this. The first time I served this to guests they couldn't believe it was just bananas. They were sure there was sugar and cream in it. This is quick to make, delicious, and you can eat it as is and be happy. Just be sure to always have some frozen bananas in a sealed container in your freezer ready to go. You can easily turn this into one of the many ice cream flavours (see below). You can also drizzle your ice cream with one of the sauces provided in the Basics section, such as chocolate, caramel, peanut butter caramel, blueberry or raspberry. How good is that?!

Serves 2

INGREDIENTS

2-3 **overripe bananas**, frozen *(bananas should definitely be soft and covered in brown spots before freezing)*

INSTRUCTIONS

1. Peel and cut bananas in to one-inch chunks. Place in sealed container or Ziploc bag in the freezer until use.
2. Put frozen bananas in food processor (or high-speed blender) and process until you have creamy, "soft serve" ice cream!
3. Serve immediately or transfer to a container, freezer for about 30 minutes and then use an ice cream scoop to serve.
4. Enjoy as is, or top with one of the many sauces found in the Basics section, such as chocolate, raspberry or caramel. Or, turn this ice cream into one of following flavours.

WAYS YOU CAN ADAPT OR ENHANCE THIS RECIPE

Optional Banana Soft Serve Ice Cream Flavours—just add one of the following:
- *Peanut Butter*—(a crowd favourite) add 3-4 T. peanut butter (or almond butter) (Note: contains nuts).
- *Vanilla*—add ½ tsp. vanilla powder or paste (or scrape inside a vanilla bean) or 1 tsp. pure vanilla extract, or more to taste.
- *Strawberry*—add 8-10 frozen strawberries to the processing.
- *Chocolate*—add 1-2 T. cocoa powder and 1 T. honey (or choice of healthy sweetener).
- *Maple Walnut*—stir in ¼ cup of roasted, chopped walnuts and 1 T. pure maple syrup.
- *Cookies & Cream*—add ¼ cup very cold coconut cream (the solid part of a can of coconut milk) to the processing. Stir in pieces of your favourite cookie. (Refrigerate the can of full-fat coconut milk overnight—the coconut cream will solidify, making it easy to remove.)
- *Mint Chocolate Chip*—add 3 or 4 drops pure peppermint extract. Stir in cacao nibs (or dark chocolate chips).
- *Coconut Ice Cream*—add ¼ - ½ cup coconut to the processing and garnish with toasted coconut.
- *Butter Pecan*—add ½ tsp. vanilla, and stir in ¼ cup roasted, chopped pecans and ¼ cup of your favourite Caramel Sauce (p.131-133), chilled...or drizzle the caramel sauce on top when serving.
- *Pistachio*—stir in ¼ cup chopped pistachios (& 2 T. pistachio butter, if you have some).
- *Fruit*—add ½ cup any frozen fruit, such as raspberries, blueberries, mango, pineapple, peach.
- *Pumpkin Pie*—add ½ tsp. pumpkin pie spice and 1-2 T. pure pumpkin puree.
- *Green Smoothie*—add a few frozen strawberries, a handful of fresh or frozen chopped spinach, and 1 T. hemp hearts.

Optional Toppings:
- Make a chocolate ice cream Sunday with our quick and easy Simple Chocolate Sauce (p.135). Or drizzle on one of the Caramel Sauces (p.131-133). After that sprinkle with cacao nibs, chocolate chips, toasted chopped almonds (or pecans, pistachios, hazelnuts etc.), fresh fruit or coconut. Or all of the above!
- Be creative. And definitely have fun!

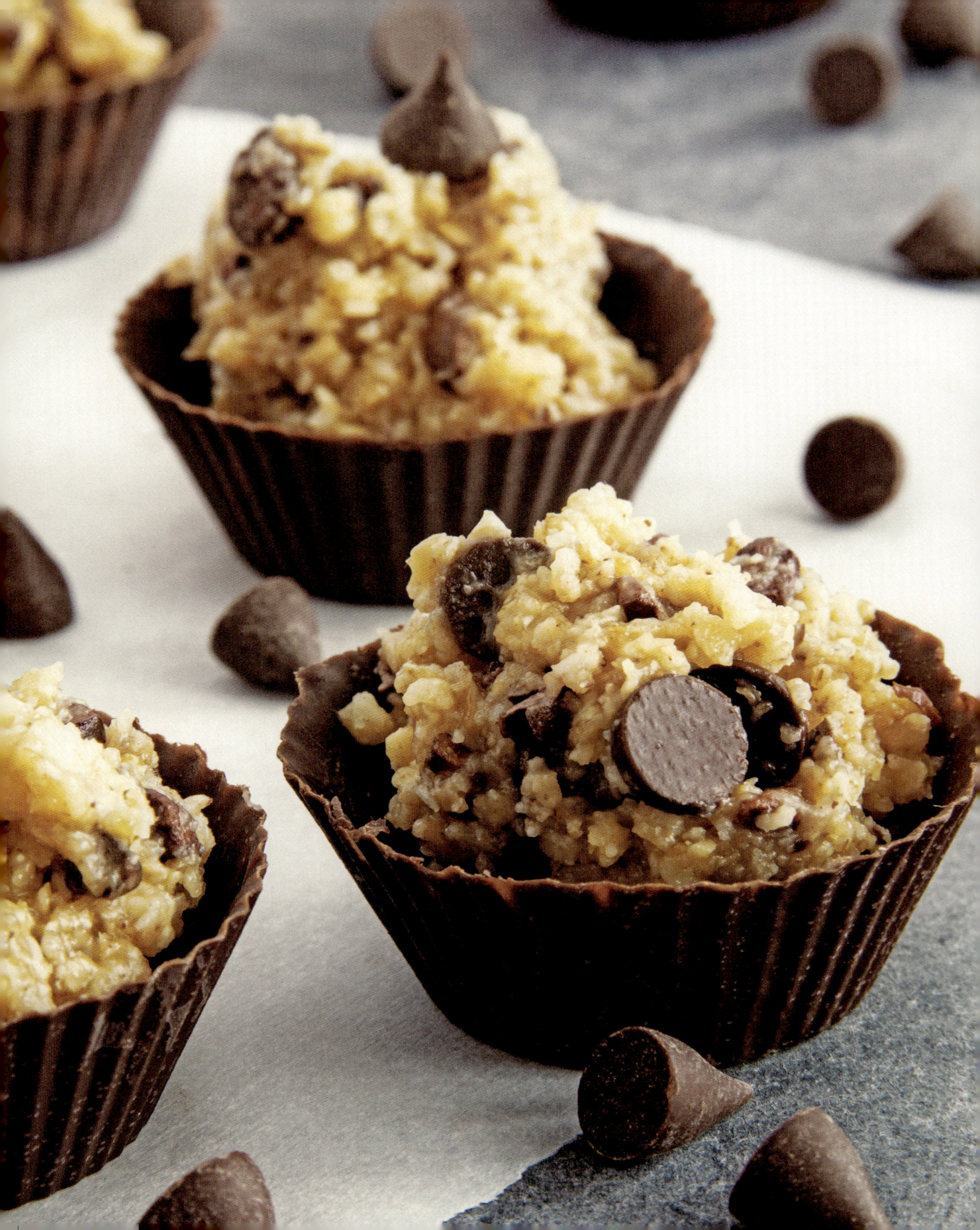

Chocolate Chip COOKIE DOUGH

IN CHOCOLATE CUPS

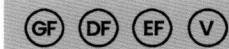

OMG, these are good! They surprised me how delicious they were the first time I created them. And they really do taste like raw cookie dough. Yet they are vegan and actually good for you! They are easy to make, and even more fun to eat! Everyone seems to love them. Just pop one of these in your mouth for a decadent, yet guilt-free treat! They are filled with protein, fibre, vitamins, minerals, healthy fats, and the best antioxidant out there: raw chocolate (cacao nibs).
Kids of all ages will love these little treats!

INGREDIENTS

12 prepared **Mini Chocolate Cups** (p.120)
¾ cup **raw cashews**
½ cup + 1 T. **rolled oats**
3 T. **unsweetened, finely-shredded coconut**
1½ T. **virgin coconut oil**, melted *(or use grass-fed butter or homemade ghee)*
3 T. **mild-tasting creamy honey**
(or pure maple syrup or coconut nectar)
1½ tsp. **pure vanilla extract**
2 pinches **sea salt**
¼ cup **bittersweet chocolate chips** *(or cacao nibs)*

INSTRUCTIONS

Make mini chocolate cups and let set in fridge 20-30 minutes while preparing the cookie dough.
1. Place cashews in food processor. Grind the cashews until they form a fine meal.
2. Add the oatmeal and coconut; pulse until it all resembles coarse meal.
3. In small saucepan, gently melt coconut oil and honey.
4. Add melted coconut oil, honey, vanilla and salt to food processor. Process until mixture creates a ball of "cookie dough". (If mixture is a little dry, add additional melted coconut oil, adding 1 tsp. at a time.)
5. Add chocolate chips and pulse 3 or 4 times to distribute evenly.
6. To assemble, portion cookie dough into 12 and place into chocolate cups.
7. Store in a sealed container.

WAYS YOU CAN ADAPT OR ENHANCE THIS RECIPE

• Garnish ideas: If you have leftover chocolate from making the chocolate cups, you can reheat it and drizzle over the filled cups. Or sprinkle each with a few cacao nibs or a pinch of shredded coconut.
• Substitute chocolate chips with raisins, dried cranberries, white chocolate chips, chopped walnuts or pecans. Or add 1-2 T. chopped, roasted almonds, walnuts, macadamias or pecans to cookie dough mixture.
• You can omit the chocolate cups and just make the cookie dough into balls and place in mini cupcake liners.
• Try omitting the chocolate chips and instead wrap cookie dough around a whole roasted macadamia nut—rolling it into a ball.

Chocolate POPCORN

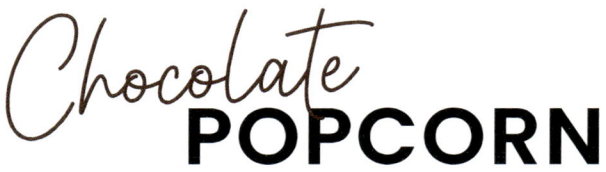

What's not to like? Popcorn AND chocolate. Hellooo!

Makes 3 cups

INGREDIENTS
3 cups **popped popcorn** *(about 2 T. unpopped kernels)*
½ cup **dark chocolate** *(preferably bittersweet, 70-85% cacao)*

INSTRUCTIONS
1. Pop the popcorn and place into large bowl or onto a parchment-lined cookie sheet. Remove any unpopped kernels.
2. Melt the chocolate slowly in a bain marie (in a bowl over simmering water— don't let bowl touch water) until chocolate is melted.
3. Drizzle melted chocolate evenly over the 3 cups of popcorn mixture. Toss gently to coat the mixture.
4. Put in the fridge to cool for about 20 minutes.

WAYS YOU CAN ADAPT OR ENHANCE THIS RECIPE
- *This is delicious on its own...and it can also be mixed with a batch of Caramel Corn (p.104), with or without nuts.*
- *If you like salted chocolate, you can sprinkle on a pinch or two of fleur de sel or flaked sea salt before refrigerating.*

Kids! Draw your favourite **dessert** here!
Of course ask your parents, first.

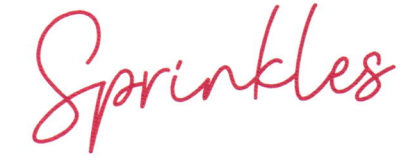

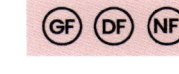

Purchased sprinkles seem harmless—they are so tiny. How could they be unhealthy? Yet they are loaded with refined sugar! They also contain corn syrup, thickeners, corn syrup, various artificial food colorings, and get this...a wax coating! Who eats wax?! My good friend Susan passed this recipe on to me. These sprinkles are made with unsweetened coconut and colored with healthy ingredients. These pretty little gems look amazing on frosted cakes and cupcakes (check out Flourless Chocolate Cupcakes with Sugarless Chocolate Frosting p.45). Have fun with them—sprinkle them on whatever you like!

INGREDIENTS

¼ cup **unsweetened shredded coconut**
For each colour:
Pink – ¼ cup **raspberries** *(fresh or frozen)*, squeezed through a strainer – use the juice
Purple – ¼ cup **blueberries** *(fresh or frozen)*, squeezed through a strainer – use the juice
Green – ¼ tsp. **spirulina powder** mixed with 1-2 T. of water
Yellow – ½ tsp. **turmeric powder** mixed with 1-2 T. of water

INSTRUCTIONS

1. Put out 4 small bowls. Add the 4 liquids separately into the 4 bowls.
2. Add ¼ cup of shredded coconut to each bowl. Mix well so all coconut is coloured.
3. Then place all of them in their respective colours onto a solid sheet, spread it around a bit and placed in the dehydrator for 3-4 hours at 115° F. degrees until completely dried.
4. Be sure they are fully dried and cooled before storing in small, sealed canning jars.

Kids! Draw cupcakes with sprinkles here!
Of course ask your parents, first.

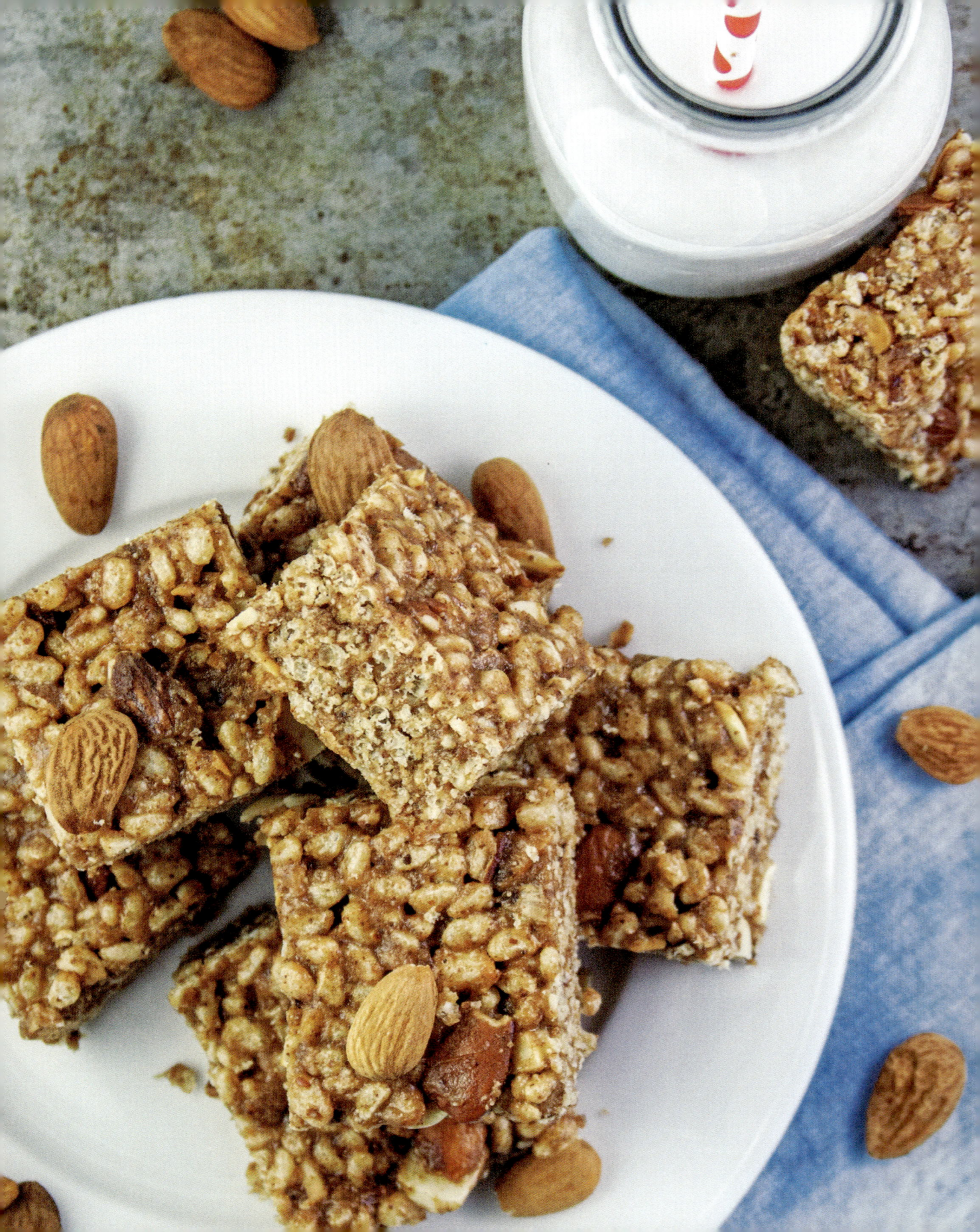

Toasted Almonds 'n Honey RICE CRISPY SQUARES

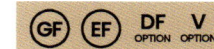

No-bake, one-bowl recipe, 4 ingredients, quick and easy, vegan... And, perfect for breakfast!
Think nut butter and cereal...how perfect for a breakfast on the run!

Makes 8x8" pan

CRUST

¾ cup **raw almonds**, roughly chopped
1 cup **almond butter** *(see Tips)*
½ cup **honey** *(for V: use alternative sweetener such as coconut nectar)*
2 cups **crispy rice cereal** *(I use organic by Nature's Path)*

Optional: 1 T. butter or homemade ghee *(for V: use vegan butter)*

CRUST INSTRUCTIONS

1. Roast chopped almonds in 350° F oven for 10-13 minutes.
2. Place nut butter and honey (and butter or ghee, if using) in saucepan and warm gently to runny consistency, 1-2 minutes.
3. Place crispy rice cereal and roasted almonds in large bowl. Pour the warm almond butter and honey mixture over top. Stir until well mixed.
4. Press firmly into 8x8" pan.
5. Chill 10 minutes and cut into squares.

TIPS
- Use purchased almond butter or make your own almond butter. See Pecan Rice Crispy Triangles (p.39) for method.
- Check honey resource on p. 12 for delicious, mild-tasting, creamy raw honey. It's 100% pure Canadian, well-priced, and they deliver.

WAYS YOU CAN ADAPT OR ENHANCE THIS RECIPE
- Substitute the almonds and almond butter with peanuts and peanut butter for a nice PB & Honey treat.
- Drizzle melted, dark chocolate on top or dip half of each square in melted chocolate and let set on parchment paper; chill in fridge.

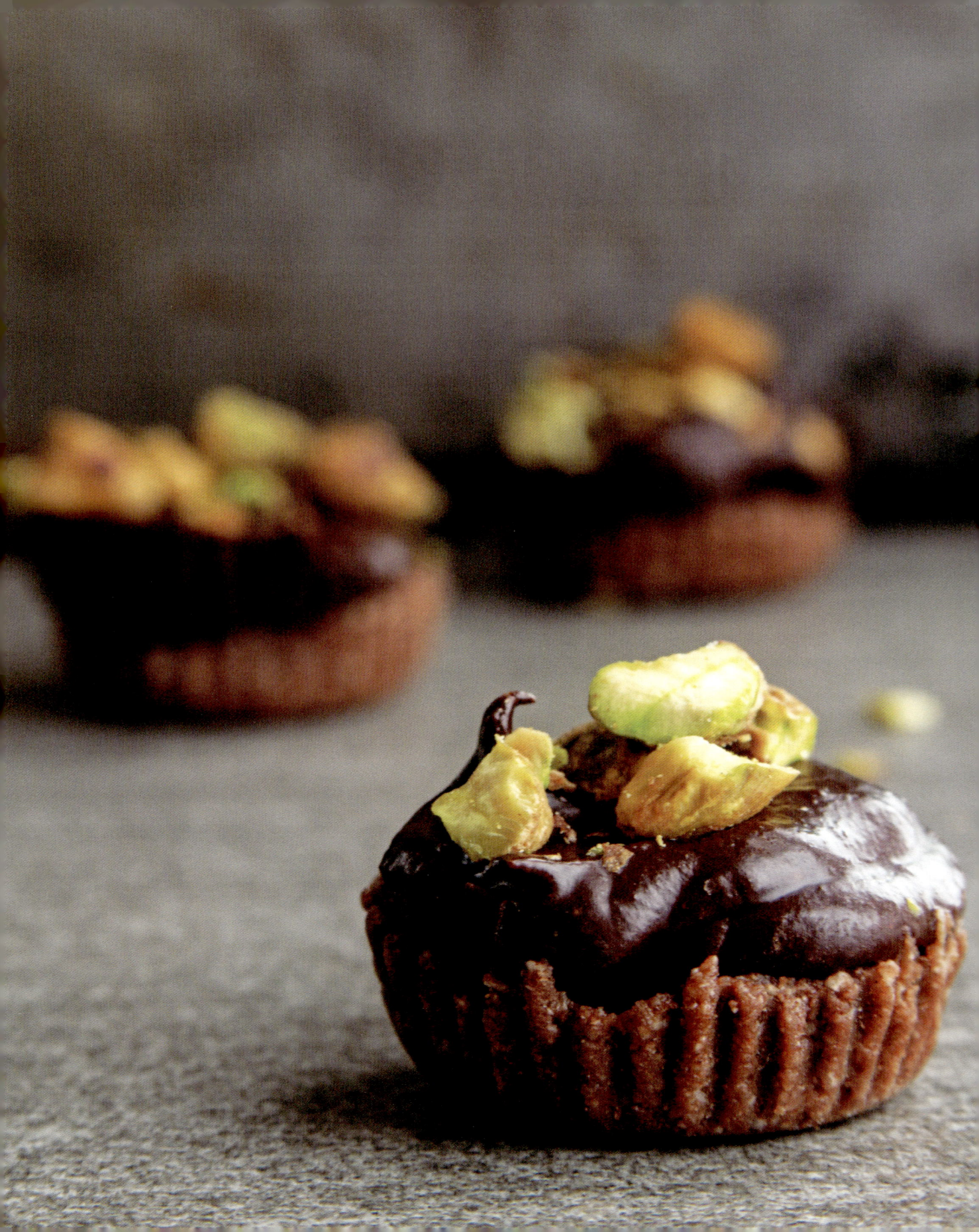

Double Chocolate Fudge MINI TARTS

GF DF EF V P

Who doesn't like a two-bite chocolate treat?! These little chocolate morsels are absolutely delicious and very easy to make. They are just the right balance between the granular base layer and the velvety-smooth chocolate ganache layer.

Makes 22-24 mini tarts

CRUST
1 cup plus 2 T. **almond flour** *(or other finely ground raw nut such as pecans, walnuts or hazelnuts)*
¼ cup **unsweetened finely-shredded coconut**
3 T. good quality **cacao powder** *(preferably raw organic)*
2 T. pure **maple syrup**
¼ cup **virgin coconut oil,** melted
⅛ tsp. **fine sea salt**

FILLING
½ cup **virgin coconut oil**, melted
⅓ cup **pure maple syrup**
1 cup **cacao powder** *(preferably raw, organic)*
Optional: ½ tsp. pure vanilla extract and pinch sea salt

INSTRUCTIONS
1. **CRUST**: In large bowl, combine first 3 ingredients with fork so there are no lumps. Add next 3 ingredients and blend well with fork.
2. Place 24 mini cupcake liners (paper or silicone) into a mini muffin/cupcake pan. Divide dough evenly among the tarts. Press dough evenly and firmly into the bottom. Chill pan until filling is prepared.
3. Prepare toppings at this point, if using.
4. **FILLING:** Add the 3 filling ingredients to large bowl and whisk well to blend until smooth and light.
5. Pour or spoon the chocolate filling into the crusts and spread evenly.
6. If adding topping, do so immediately after filling.
7. Refrigerate tarts to set and firm for 1-2 hours. Store in sealed container in fridge for up to a week.
Note: They soften quickly at room temperature.

WAYS YOU CAN ADAPT OR ENHANCE THIS RECIPE
- Topping Ideas: Sprinkle a small amount of one of these toppings on each tartlet before refrigerating: shelled pistachios, walnut half, almond, pecan half, chocolate chips, shredded coconut, hemp seeds, edible flower, pinch of flaked sea salt, or a drizzle of melted white or milk chocolate.
- Alternate fillings:
  - Use 1 cup of homemade Nutella (Hazel-Nut-Ella Chocolate Spread, p.144) at room temperature. Spoon about 2 tsp. into each cup and spread out to create a top layer. Top with a roasted hazelnut.
  - For "Chocolate Mint" tartlets, add ½ tsp. good quality peppermint extract to the filling.
  - Add 1 cup crispy rice cereal to filling.

BASICS

Caramel Sauces *131-133*

Chocolate Sauces, Ganache & Frosting *134-136*

Easy Oil Pie Crust *137*

Spelt & Butter Shortbread Crust *138*

Pecan Oat Crust *139*

"Graham" Crust *139*

Butter-Vinegar Shortbread Pie Crust *140*

Caramelized Apples *141*

Raspberry Coulis *142*

Blueberry Sauce *(cooked & raw versions)* *142*

Date Paste *143*

Pecan Praline Butter *143*

Hazel-Nut-Ella Chocolate Spread *(homemade "Nutella")* *144*

Lemon Curd made with Honey *145*

No-Cook Fruit Jam *146*

Almond Milk *147*

Cashew Milk & Cashew Creams *148*

Oat Milk *149*

CARAMEL SAUCES

Also called dulce de leche, these caramel sauces are to die for. I admit—caramel sauce is a weakness of mine! I have been known to just eat it with a spoon. J I also love it on all the things that you might have caramel sauce on! Think cheesecakes (see p.63 and p.69)—just heat gently and drizzle on each piece when serving. Or drizzle on Banana Soft Serve Ice Cream (p.121) or Fudgy Butternut Squash Espresso Brownies (p.77). Perhaps try in a Caramel Latté (p.98), or as a decadent and sweet filling in Chocolate Cups with Fillings (p.120). Or use in Caramel Pecan Banana Tarts (p.65) or Turtle Tarts (p.65). Turn any caramel sauce in to salted caramel—see recipe #8. What I also really like for a quick, sweet snack or dessert is fresh fruit dipped into caramel sauce (pieces of banana, apple, pear, strawberries). See also Fruit on a Stick (p.119). Unlike some caramel sauces made with refined white or brown sugar, these are all quick to make and healthier options. (These are all gluten-free, refined sugar-free, and some even dairy-free!) My fave is #1 but I like all the variations! *Store caramel sauces in sealed jar in fridge for up to two weeks.*

1. Almond Butter CARAMEL SAUCE

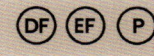

Makes just over 1 cup

INGREDIENTS
½ cup **pure maple syrup**
¼ cup **grass-fed butter** or **homemade ghee**
½ cup **creamy almond butter**
½ tsp. **pure vanilla extract**
pinch **sea salt**

INSTRUCTIONS
1. In a medium saucepan, heat maple syrup and butter until butter is just melted. Remove from heat and add rest of the ingredients (almond butter, vanilla, salt). Whisk until well combined. (Note: If your almond butter is thick, you may need less. Start with less and add until you get a consistency you like.)
2. Store in sealed container. Caramel sauce will thicken in the fridge—so enjoy as is, or reheat gently in a saucepan.

2. One Bowl CARAMEL SAUCE

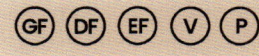

Makes 1 cup

INGREDIENTS
2 T. **coconut butter** *(or homemade ghee, slowly melted)*
1 T. melted **coconut oil** *(or grass-fed butter, if you prefer)*
½ cup **pure maple syrup**
3 T. **creamy almond butter** *(or cashew butter)*
2 T. **lucuma powder** *(sifted to reduce lumps)*
1½ tsp. **pure vanilla extract**
2 pinches **sea salt**

INSTRUCTIONS
1. Slowly melt coconut butter in bowl over simmering water. Add coconut oil near the end.
2. Remove from heat and add rest of ingredients and whisk until smooth.
3. Store in sealed container in fridge for up to two weeks.

3. Butter & Coconut Sugar CARAMEL SAUCE

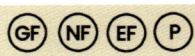

Makes 1¼ cups

INGREDIENTS
½ cup **grass-fed butter** (*or homemade ghee—see Tips*)
¾ cup **coconut sugar**
2 T. **water**
2 T. **coconut cream** (*the solid part from a can of full-fat coconut milk*)
1 tsp. **pure vanilla extract**
¼ tsp. **sea salt**

INSTRUCTIONS
1. Combine caramel sauce ingredients in a small saucepan and heat until butter is melted, stirring occasionally. After mixture is smooth and well combined, continue stirring to allow caramel to thicken, about 3-5 minutes.
2. Remove caramel from heat and set aside until use. Store in sealed container in fridge. Caramel sauce will thicken in the fridge—so enjoy as is, or reheat gently in a saucepan.

TIPS
This caramel sauce isn't dairy-free, but you could use homemade ghee in place of butter, if you are concerned about the small amount of dairy in butter.

4. Spiced CARAMEL SAUCE

Add any of the following spice combinations to any of the above caramel sauces:
- ½ tsp. **cinnamon**, ¼ tsp. **ginger**, and a pinch of **cloves**, **sea salt** and **vanilla powder**
- ¼ tsp. each of **cloves**, **cinnamon**, **black pepper** and **anise**
- ½ tsp. **cardamom**, ¼ tsp. each of **ginger** and **cinnamon**

...add more or less spice, to taste

5. Peanut Butter CARAMEL SAUCE

Makes 1¼ cups

Use one batch of either **#1 Almond Butter Caramel Sauce** or **#2 One-Bowl Caramel** Sauce and substitute the almond butter with **creamy peanut butter**. Then add an additional ¼ cup of **peanut butter** and whisk to blend well.

6. Pumpkin Spice CARAMEL SAUCE

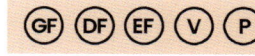

Makes approx. 1¼ cups

INGREDIENTS

½ cup **pure maple syrup**
⅓ cup **creamy almond butter**
⅓ cup **virgin coconut oil**
3 T. **unsweetened pumpkin puree** *(not pumpkin pie mix)*
2 tsp. **vanilla extract**
1-2 tsp. **pumpkin pie spice**
(see p.58 to make up own pumpkin pie spice mixture)
¼ tsp. **sea salt**

INSTRUCTIONS

1. Vigorously whisk together all ingredients in a saucepan over medium-low heat until mixture is smooth and slightly thickened, about 3 minutes.
2. Remove from heat and enjoy warm, or let cool to thicken.
3. Store in sealed container in fridge. Caramel sauce will thicken in the fridge—so enjoy as is, or reheat gently in a saucepan.

7. Boozy CARAMEL SAUCE

Whiskey is a natural addition to Caramel Sauce. Using **Caramel Sauce #1, 2 or 3**, add 1 T. of **whiskey or bourbon**. Or add 2-3 T. of **liqueur**, such as Amaretto. Or add rum and use to drizzle on Baked Coconut Eggnog Custard (p.51).
Be sure to mix choice of alcohol in at the end—do not heat.

8. Salted CARAMEL SAUCE

Turn any Caramel Sauce in to "Salted" Caramel Sauce by simply adding ½ - 1 tsp. sea salt to caramel mixture (to taste). I suggest using **Caramel Sauce #1, 2 or 3** to make "salted".
I prefer to sprinkle **flaked sea salt** (such as Maldon) **or fleur de sel** on top when serving.

GF EF P DF OPTION NF OPTION V OPTION

CHOCOLATE SAUCES, GANACHE & FROSTING

These sauces can be used to make hot chocolate, served over ice cream (duh!) or drizzled over almost anything in this book (wink, wink). Try over Peanut Butter Swirl Protein Bars (p.25), Fudgy Butternut Squash Espresso Brownies (p.77), Caramel Pecan Banana Tarts (p.65), Pecan Rice Crispy Triangles (p.39), Chocolate Chip Cookie Dough in Chocolate Cups (p.123), Baked Cashew Cheesecake (p.69) or Banana Soft Serve Ice Cream (p.121). Perhaps use as a dip for fresh or dried fruit pieces (think strawberries, banana, apple, dried apricots) or dip Apple Chips (p.110) or Fudgsicles (p.107) in warm chocolate sauce and let them firm up in freezer. Or, if you're like me...dip your spoon right in and enjoy a mouthful of chocolate heaven! Consider a Boozy version of the Chocolate sauces by adding a small amount of whiskey or bourbon, or your favourite liqueur, such as orange, hazelnut or almond.
Or stir in ½ tsp. freshly grated orange zest for an orange-chocolate sauce.

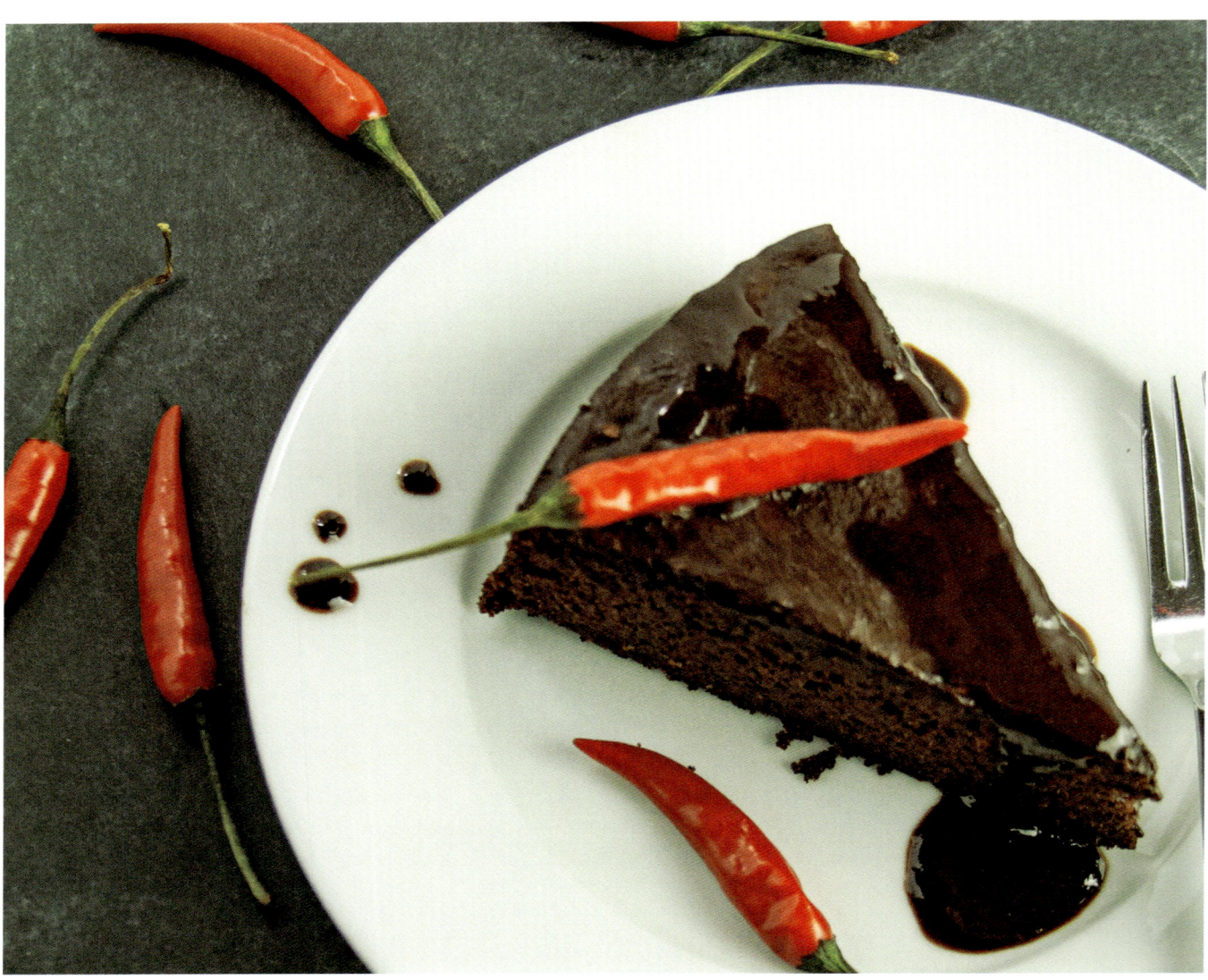

1. Simple CHOCOLATE SAUCE

GF DF NF EF V P

A Hot Fudge Sauce when warm! An easy, quick and delicious chocolate sauce that takes 2 minutes to make. Why would you ever want to buy chocolate sauce in a jar again?!
Note: If you happen to have leftovers, this sauce will solidify; simply reheat to liquefy.

INGREDIENTS

¼ cup **good quality cacao powder** *(preferably raw, organic)*
2 T. **pure maple syrup** *(add up to 2 more T. if you like a sweeter sauce)*
2 T. **virgin coconut oil**, or **homemade ghee**

INSTRUCTIONS

1. Place all ingredients in small saucepan over medium-low heat, whisking while it's heating to blend ingredients. (Optional: add ¼ tsp. vanilla and pinch of salt.)
2. Store in a sealed jar in fridge for 1-2 weeks.

2. Almond Butter CHOCOLATE SAUCE

GF DF EF V P

This is so delicious. It's creamy and rich, yet not too sweet. This is another recipe that is so easy to make. The sauce will harden slightly when refrigerated; to liquify, simply reheat gently in a saucepan.

INGREDIENTS

1 T. **virgin coconut oil**, melted *(or homemade ghee)*
3 T. **pure maple syrup**
2 T. good quality **cacao powder** *(preferably raw, organic)*
1 T. **almond butter**, or cashew butter
½ tsp. **pure vanilla extract**
pinch **sea salt**
1 T. **warm water**

INSTRUCTIONS

1. Place all ingredients in a medium-sized bowl and whisk until smooth.
2. Store in a sealed jar in the fridge for 1-2 weeks.

3. Chocolate Chili GANACHE

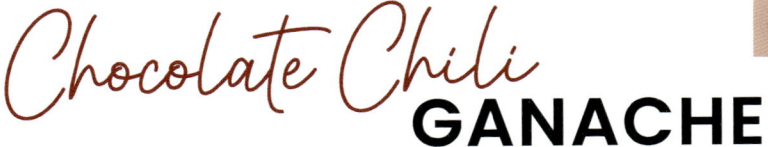

Makes ½ cup

Okay, this is an absolutely delicious chocolate ganache with a subtle spicy bite...a sauce that was originally created for the Chocolate & Chili Quinoa Cake (p.81), inspired by Mexican hot chocolate flavours. I also discovered that the leftovers were amazing used in other ways. I added coconut milk to the leftovers and voila—I created a nice rich, creamy Mexican type Hot Chocolate (see p.100). Yum!

INGREDIENTS
¼ cup **virgin coconut oil** *(or butter or homemade ghee)*
¼ cup good quality **cacao powder** *(preferably raw, organic)*
¼ cup **pure maple syrup**
½ tsp. **pure vanilla extract**
pinch **sea salt**
¼ tsp. each of **ancho chili powder, cinnamon & cayenne** *(use less cayenne if you prefer less heat)*

INSTRUCTIONS
1. Place all ingredients in small saucepan over medium-low heat, whisking while it's heating to blend ingredients. Remove from heat and cool to room temperature about 10-15 minutes if using on the Chocolate & Chili Quinoa Cake (p.81).
2. Store in a sealed jar in the fridge for 1-2 weeks.

4. Sugarless CHOCOLATE FROSTING

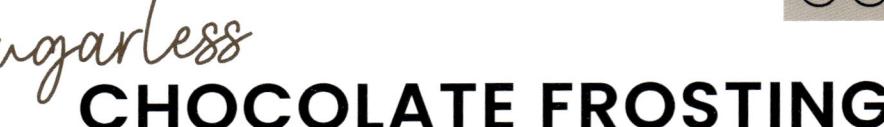

Yes, frosting can be healthy! Look at these pure ingredients. Never go without frosting a cake or cupcake when you can have this. It's sugarless, dairy-free and absolute chocolatey goodness. Use this to top Flourless Chocolate Cupcakes (p.45), Chocolate & Chili Quinoa Cake with Chocolate-Chili Ganache (p.81), Flourless Chocolate Cake (p.86), or fill Mini Chocolate Cups (p.120).

INGREDIENTS
1 large, perfectly ripe **avocado**, pitted, peeled, and roughly chopped
½ cup good quality **cacao powder, sifted** *(preferably raw, organic)*
½ cup **pure maple syrup**
½ tsp. **pure vanilla extract**
pinch fine **sea salt**

INSTRUCTIONS
1. Blend all ingredients in a food processor until it's very smooth and creamy. Stop to scrape down sides occasionally, if necessary.
2. Frosting is ready to use... or place in fridge to firm up, if you like. Or add a little water if it's too thick.

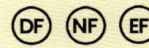

Easy OIL PIE CRUST

This is my go-to pie crust. It is not only easy to make (no laborious cutting in of butter or lard) but is amazingly still flakey and tender like a crust should be. This is healthier version, of course, with a healthy oil of your choice! Just stir these ingredients in a bowl and voila!...ready to roll out. So simple! I have tried various flours and they don't turn out as well as white—so this is one of the few recipes in the cookbook where I use all-purpose white flour. However, I have used spelt flour and it is also good. I use this crust for sweet and savory pies and tarts. This recipe makes 2 thin crusts. If you only need one pie crust, consider making the full batch anyways and making a few tarts (i.e. Lemon Tarts, p.67) with the leftover dough. Or roll out the extra dough and use cookie cutters to make shapes to place on top of your pie for decoration. Or simply place them on a lined cookie sheet and bake separately until golden brown.

Makes approximately 2 bottom pie crusts or one 9" double pie crust or several mini tarts
(it all depends on how thin you roll the dough and the size of your pie/tart pans)

INGREDIENTS

1¾ cups **all-purpose flour** *(preferably organic, white, unbleached)*

1 tsp. **fine sea salt**

½ cup **oil** *(use mild-flavoured oil such as avocado, grapeseed or sunflower)*

¼ cup **ice-cold milk or water** *(for V: use plant-based milk of choice)*

INSTRUCTIONS

1. Preheat oven to 400° F. (You will be baking at 350° F.)
2. With a fork, mix flour and salt together in a medium-sized bowl.
3. Stir in oil until blended.
4. Stir in ice-cold milk.
5. Work dough with hands, if necessary, to form a ball.
6. Use ½-¾ of dough between 2 layers of plastic wrap or parchment paper.
7. If blind baking (pre-baking) pie shell, for such recipes as Lemon Tarts (p.67) or Fresh Raspberry Pie (p. 53), poke several holes into bottom and sides of crust with a fork, and bake 350° F for 12-16 minutes or until fully cooked and lightly golden.
8. If using for a pie that bakes, such as Apple Tart Pie (p.47), Pumpkin Pie (p.58), or Maple Syrup Pie (p.64), refrigerate until pie filling is ready. Or you can parbake (partially bake) it for 7-10 minutes at 350° F, if you prefer.

TIPS

- Be sure the milk (or water) is ice-cold (use ice cube in water). This will result in a flakier crust.
- I roll out dough between two pieces of plastic wrap, to make handling easier. I roll quite thin because I like a thin pie crust, but you can choose your pie crust thickness to suit you.
- Wrap unused portion of pastry with plastic wrap until ready to use. Or create cut-outs to bake separately and place on pie after baking.
- Baking time will vary depending on the thickness of your crust. Pie crust can burn quickly so watch carefully. Note that most pie crusts (including this one) shrink when baked.
- If you want to use spelt flour, then add less liquids. Let me know if you find a GF flour that works well in this recipe.

Spelt & Butter SHORTBREAD CRUST

This is a grainy, crispy crust that bursts with flavour. It's hearty, a bit nutty-flavoured and is sturdy—it bodes well to holding a heavier filling, such as Fresh Raspberry Pie (p.53), Apple Tart Pie (p.47), Pumpkin Pie (p.58) and Baked Cashew Cheesecake (p.69)... or any tart or pie you desire. Spelt is not gluten-free, but it has less gluten than wheat and it is easier to digest than wheat. It is an ancient grain and has not been modified from its natural state and is higher in fibre and nutrition. Spelt often substitutes well 1:1 for white and whole wheat flour. Adapted from "Everyday Pie".

Makes one large pie crust (or six 3½" tarts)

INGREDIENTS

1½ cups *(180 g)* **whole grain spelt flour**
1 T. **coconut sugar**
¼ tsp. **sea salt**
¼ tsp. **baking powder**
10 T. *(140g)* **grass-fed butter**, cut in small cubes
2 T. *(30g)* **cream cheese**, cut in small cubes *(or substitute with 2 more T. butter)*
¼ cup ice-cold **water**

INSTRUCTIONS

1. In a food processor, pulse together spelt flour, sugar, salt and baking powder until combined.
2. Add butter and pulse 8 short bursts.
3. Add cream cheese and pulse 4 more times.
4. Pour the ice-cold water in the chute with motor running, and pulse just until the dough forms a ball.
5. This moist dough lends itself well to pressing the dough to fit the pan. I like to first roll the dough thinly between 2 sheets of plastic wrap and then "push" the rest into the pan. (There may be leftover dough—see Tips.)
6. If using it with a baked filling, such as Apple Tart Pie (p.47), Maple Syrup Pie (p.64) or Pumpkin Pie (p.58), then poke several holes in crust with a fork and parbake it at 400° F. for 10-15 minutes first, before filling and baking. If blind baking this crust (baking without a filling) such as for Fresh Raspberry Pie (p.53) or Lemon Tarts (p. 67), poke several holes into the crust, then line the crust with parchment paper or foil that overhangs the rim and fill with pie weights or dried beans or rice). Bake in preheated 350° F. oven for about 20 minutes. Remove parchment and pie weights and bake another 10 minutes, or until crust is golden brown and bottom is cooked through.
Note: If not using the dough immediately, form the dough in to a ball and wrap it tightly in plastic and refrigerate for up to 48 hours. (Or freeze for later.)

TIPS

• *This recipe makes enough for a large pie crust (i.e. 11" pie pan, or 13" glass tart pan) so you may have leftovers if you like a thinner pie crust or are using a smaller pie pan. Use the leftover dough to create decorative cut-outs to place on the pie. (I bake them on a parchment lined cookie sheet separately and then arrange them on the pie after baking, but depending on the pie, you can bake the decorations on the pie.)*
• *Measure flour, cream cheese and butter by weight, if you possibly can—it makes for more accurate results.*

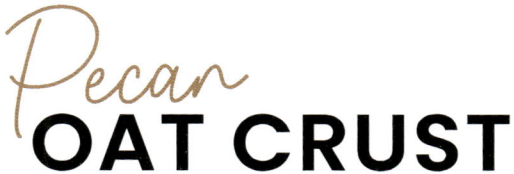

Pecan OAT CRUST

EF OPTION · GF OPTION · DF OPTION · V OPTION

This is delicious and super easy (no rolling) crust for pies and tarts. It's a push-in crust—no rolling! The nutty pecan flavour combined with the oatmeal is a nice change from the traditional pie crust. You can use this recipe in place of any traditional pie crust (for bottom crust pies only). Make in food processor, press into a pie pan and bake. Feel free to try other nuts in place of the pecans, such as almonds, hazelnuts or walnuts.

Makes crust for one 8-9" pie, or five or six 3" removable bottom tarts

INGREDIENTS

½ cup **raw pecans**
1¼ cup **rolled oats** *(or quick oats) (for GF: use gluten-free oats)*
¼ cup **unsalted butter**, melted *(for DF & V: use coconut oil, avocado oil, or 2 T. of each)*
2 T. **honey** *(for V: use pure maple syrup, coconut nectar, or ¼ cup soft medjool dates)*
½ tsp. **fine sea salt**

For Chocolate Pecan Oat Crust, add 2-3 T. of cacao powder to step #2. If it becomes too dry, just add a little more butter or oil.

INSTRUCTIONS

1. Preheat oven to 350° F.
2. In food processor, blend pecans until roughly chopped. Add oats and process until a fine crumble.
3. Add in butter, honey and salt and process until well combined and ball forms.
4. Press mixture into bottom of a 9-inch pie pan (removable bottom or springform pan).
5. Bake 15-20 minutes (for tarts bake about 10 minutes), or until crust is cooked through and nicely browned.
6. Remove from oven and cool completely on cooling rack before filling.

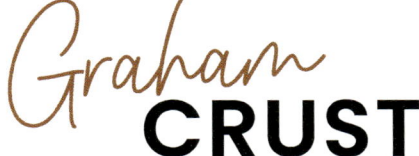

Graham CRUST

GF · DF · EF · V OPTION

A healthy version of a graham cracker crust—no refined sugar and other undesired ingredients. Unlike a purchased graham cracker crust, this version is gluten-free and flour-free.

Same recipe as above but substitute honey with
1 T. molasses, and add ¼ tsp. cinnamon.

TIPS

• *Fill either of these cooked pie crusts with your favourite filling. Try Fresh Raspberry Pie with Raspberry-Honey Glaze (p.53), or make a lemon pie using Lemon Curd made with Honey (p. 145) as your filling.*
• *Use for a baked filling such as Baked Cashew Cheesecake (p. 69)—just fill and bake per recipe instructions.*

Butter-Vinegar SHORTBREAD PIE CRUST

NF · EF · GF OPTION · DF OPTION · V OPTION

Okay, I admit...this is my favourite pie crust recipe because I LOVE the flavour of butter and it is prominent in this recipe. Of course, I buy the best butter possible... grass-fed/pasture-raised butter! Note—you don't taste the vinegar. It's just a secret ingredient that makes for a better, flakier crust. I also love this pastry because it is so easy to make. I make it all in the food processor, and there is no required rolling out—just push it into the pie pan. I almost exclusively use fluted, removable bottom flan pans for my pies now because they look pretty and they are easy to remove from the pan. Subsequently they are easier to cut, especially that first piece!

Makes one 9 or 10" bottom pie crust (or removable bottom flan/tart crust, or several tartlets)

INGREDIENTS

1 cup **all-purpose flour** (for GF: see Adaptations)
¼ tsp. **fine sea salt**
2 T. **maple sugar** or **coconut sugar**, finely ground (see Tips)
½ cup **cold unsalted butter**, cut into ½" cubes (if using salted butter, omit added salt)
1 T. **white vinegar**

INSTRUCTIONS

1. In food processor, combine flour, salt and sugar.
2. With food processor running, add all pieces of butter at once. Blend until mixture resembles small peas or course meal.
3. Add vinegar and pulse only until mixture is blended. (Do not over-blend!) If necessary, add 1 tsp. of ice-cold water.
4. Remove mixture from food processor; create a ball.
5. Push into pie plate, removable bottom flan pan (or tart shells). Press evenly on bottom and up sides of pan. (Note: You can roll out this pastry, if you prefer. Refrigerate plastic-wrapped ball of pastry for 20 minutes, first. Roll out between sheets of parchment or plastic wrap.)
6. At this point, refrigerate the crust in the pie pan for 30-60 minutes while making a filling for baking, such as for Apple Tart Pie (p.47), Maple Syrup Pie (p.64), or Pumpkin Pie (p.58). OR parbake (partially bake) the crust at 400° F for 20 minutes before adding the filling and returning to the oven. Poke several holes in the crust with a fork before par-baking.
7. If pre-baking (also called blind baking—meaning there is no filling) for uncooked pie fillings such as Fresh Raspberry Pie (p.53) or Lemon Tarts, (p.67), then refrigerate the crust for 1 hour or longer. Then line the crust with a piece of parchment paper or foil that overhangs rim. Fill with pie weights (or dried beans or rice). Bake at 425° F. for 15 minutes. Then reduce oven to 375° F., remove the parchment and pie weights and bake about 5 minutes longer, until crust is golden brown and bottom is cooked through. Cool to room temperature before filling.

TIPS
- *If using white flour, then try to find organic, unbleached, all-purpose flour.*
- *For fine coconut sugar, simply grind coconut sugar in a coffee grinder or blender.*

WAYS YOU CAN ADAPT OR ENHANCE THIS RECIPE
- *For a gluten-free crust, simply substitute flour with a gluten-free all-purpose flour mix—preferably a good quality, organic one. (I use Namaste or Soleil organic all-purpose GF flour mixes.) Please note the taste and texture will vary from the traditional flour crust. I sometimes substitute spelt flour for the white flour, but I sift it and use a little less. Each flour will produce slightly different results.*
- *For DF and V, substitute butter with a good quality vegan butter.*

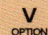

Caramelized APPLES

This is so simple to make, and delicious served on almost anything! Try on Baked Cashew Cheesecake (p.69), waffles, pancakes, hot oatmeal, breakfast power bowls, vanilla coconut ice cream, Banana Soft Serve Ice Cream (p.121) or over a banana cut in half lengthwise. Check out other fruit to caramelize below.

Makes 4 servings

INGREDIENTS
2 T. **grass-fed butter**, or **homemade ghee** (for V: use vegan butter)
2 T. **coconut sugar**
2 **apples**, peeled, cored and thinly sliced *(see Tips for best apples to use)*
pinch **sea salt**

INSTRUCTIONS
1. Melt butter over medium-high heat in large skillet.
2. Add coconut sugar and salt. Stir to combine.
3. Add apples and stir to coat. Cook for about 5-10 minutes, stirring constantly, until apples are tender.

TIPS
• Best apples to use are Granny Smith, Golden Delicious, Braeburn or Gala.
• Peeling apples is optional. The peel contains antioxidants, fibre, vitamin A, K, C and potassium, so I often keep the peels on—it's up to you.

WAYS YOU CAN ADAPT OR ENHANCE THIS RECIPE
• Other fruit that can be caramelized: bananas, pears, peaches or mangos.

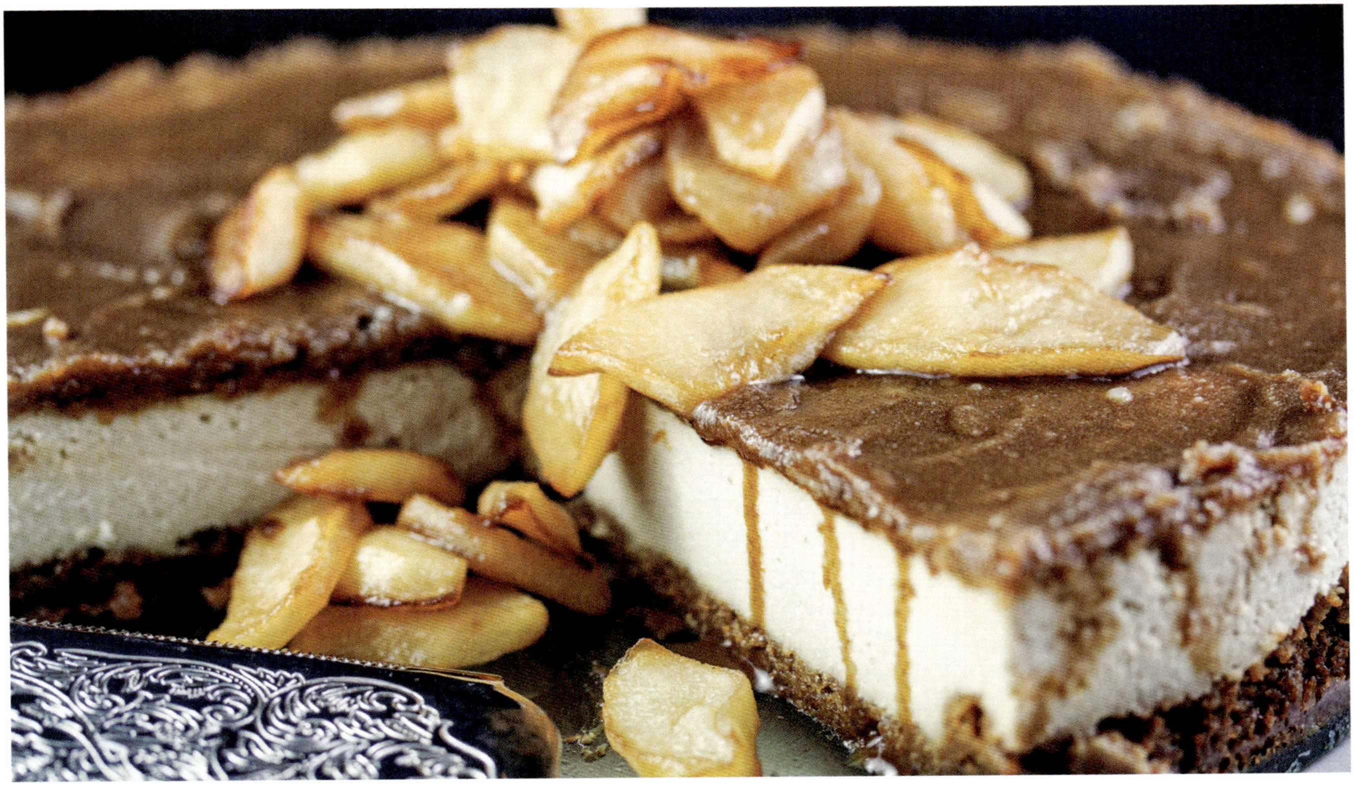

Raspberry COULIS

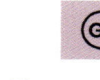 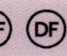   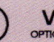

I love this sauce because it tastes so fresh! It is raw (uncooked) so you don't lose that fresh raspberry flavour. Try it drizzled over desserts such as Flourless Chocolate Cake (p.86), Berrylicious Cashew Cheesecake (p.49), Fudgy Butternut Squash Espresso Brownies (p.77), Lemon Cashew Cheesecake (p.63), or as a layer in Parfaits (p.54). Drizzle it over sliced bananas, on toast with any nut butter, or over your granola or porridge. Use it in smoothies or as a dip for pieces of fresh fruit like orange segments, banana or apple slices. Delicious drizzled on ice cream. Raspberry Coulis pairs well with chocolate so be sure to try it in Mini Chocolate Cups (p.120). Check out the chocolate section and see how much fun you will have trying some combinations!
Also try this recipe with alternate fruit—see list below.

INGREDIENTS

2 cups fresh or frozen **raspberries**
(if frozen, thaw first, and drain most of liquid. Straining is optional.)
¼ cup **honey**, to taste
(for V: use maple syrup or coconut nectar)
1-2 tsp. **fresh lemon juice** *(see adaptations below)*

INSTRUCTIONS

1. Place all ingredients in a high-speed blender for one minute. Strain through a fine-mesh sieve, using a spoon to stir and push until all the sauce is through. (Straining is optional.)
2. When ready to serve, place a few tablespoons in a small plastic bag and cut a small portion of the end to create an easy piping bag. Drizzle on cake and plate.
3. Store covered in fridge for up to a week.

WAYS YOU CAN ADAPT OR ENHANCE THIS RECIPE

- *Optional substitution for raspberries, strawberries, blackberries, mangos, peaches or kiwifruit.*
- *Substitute lemon with orange (try zest and juice of half a small orange). Or sub with 1 tsp. vanilla and a pinch of salt.*

Blueberry SAUCE

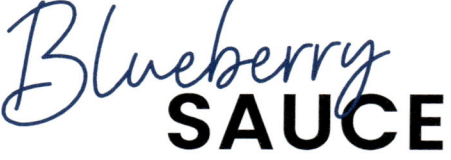 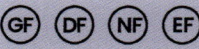 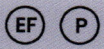 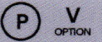

I love blueberries and blueberry sauce is no exception. Here are two variations of Blueberry Sauce; both are 3 ingredients... so simple and easy to make. I love the cooked sauce on waffles & pancakes and hot oatmeal/porridge. I love the raw sauce as a topping on Blueberry Instant Ice Cream (p.50), Banana Soft Serve Ice Cream (p.121), Coconut Chia Pudding (p.61), Baked Cashew Cheesecake (p.69), as a dip for fruit, or as a layer in a Parfait (p. 54). Both are good used as a crêpe or blintz filling.

INGREDIENTS

4 cups of **blueberries**, fresh or frozen *(thawed slightly)*
¼ cup **honey**
(for V: use pure maple syrup or coconut nectar)
1 T. **fresh lemon juice**

COOKED BLUEBERRY SAUCE:

1. Place blueberries and sweetener in medium saucepan with 1-2 T. of water.
2. Bring to boil and then simmer on medium-low until desired consistency, about 20-30 minutes.
3. Remove from heat and stir in fresh lemon juice.

RAW/UNCOOKED BLUEBERRY SAUCE:

Place all ingredients in high-speed blender and blend until smooth. (It is fine to have some lumps and texture.)

TIPS:

- *Store leftovers in sealed mason jar in fridge. Will keep for up to one week.*

WAYS YOU CAN ADAPT OR ENHANCE THIS RECIPE

- *If you like more lemon piquancy, add a teaspoon of lemon zest.*
- *You can substitute the lemon juice with pure vanilla extract, but may want to use a little less.*

Date PASTE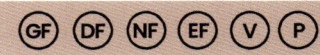

Just one ingredient—dates! Sometimes called Date Spread, this is a versatile recipe that can be used in many ways—as a sweetener in cakes, cookies, smoothies, truffles and chocolate desserts. Use this in Date Squares (p.28), or to "frost" Queen Elizabeth Date Cake (p.42). Or use it as a cookie sandwich filling, in Mini Chocolate Cups (p.120), or on toast, GF Banana Muffins (p.96), pancakes, or to sweeten smoothies. You've got to love dates—nature's candy!

Makes about 1¼ cups

INGREDIENTS
2 cups *(approx. 350 g)* **medjool** or **deglet noor dates**, pits removed, roughly chopped
2 cups **boiling water**

INSTRUCTIONS
1. Place dates in medium-sized bowl and pour hot water over top.
2. Cover the bowl with plastic wrap and let soak until dates are soft and tender. Medjool dates only need about 15 minutes. Deglet noor will need to soak for 1-2 hours.
3. Drain the dates, reserving the soaking water.
4. Place the drained dates in a food processor and process until a smooth paste. Add reserved soaking water only if you want a thinner consistency by adding 1 T. at a time to acquire the consistency you like. (Be careful not to add too much water—you don't want it runny—it should hold its shape when scooped out. I like it to have some texture, but some people like it smooth.)
5. Store in sealed jar in the fridge for up to 2 weeks.

Pecan Praline BUTTER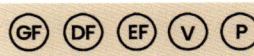

This is easy to make! Warning: Addictive...in a good way. You can omit the coconut sugar for simply "Pecan Butter" ...equally delicious.

INGREDIENTS
2 cups **raw pecans**
2 T. **coconut sugar** *(use up to 4 T. if prefer sweeter)*
1 or 2 pinches **sea salt**

INSTRUCTIONS
1. Roast all the pecans in preheated 300° F. oven for 10-12 minutes, or until they are roasted and fragrant. (They burn quickly, so watch carefully.)
2. Place roasted pecans with the other ingredients in a food processor fit with an S-blade. Process until it becomes "pecan butter"—the consistency of nut butter. This may take a few minutes, and you will need to stop occasionally to scrape down the sides.

WAYS YOU CAN ADAPT OR ENHANCE THIS RECIPE
- Can add ½ - ¾ tsp. cinnamon, ½ tsp. vanilla extract or powder, and more pinches of salt.
- Substitute coconut sugar with honey or pure maple syrup.
- If you prefer thinner consistency, choose liquid sweetener or add 1 tsp. of neutral flavoured oil to the processing.

Hazel-Nut-Ella
CHOCOLATE SPREAD
HOMEMADE "NUTELLA"

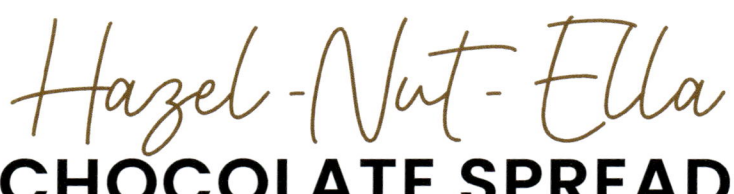

Italians love Nutella. I, too, loved it for a while, but soon realized the ingredients weren't particularly healthy. Then I discovered you can make it yourself with natural ingredients. So…I've adapted this from various recipes to come up with what I think is perfect. Everyone who has tried it loves it, and prefers it to the original Nutella. And bonus—it's guilt-free. This spread can be used cold, room temperature or heated gently. Like caramel sauce, I can eat this with a spoon. However, you can enjoy it many ways. Try spreading it on toast, sliced bananas, cookies, pizzelles, brownies, or drizzled on ice cream. Use as a tart filling. Okay, I admit, I was playing with things to do with it because I'm in love with the stuff. Try using it to make amazing Nutella Truffles (p.78), or as the filling in Nutella Chocolate Cups (p.78). You can also use it as an alternate filling for the Double Chocolate Fudge Mini Tarts (p.129). Or use it to make a chocolate smoothie, as a cookie sandwich filling, or as a dip for Apple Chips (p.110).

Makes 3 cups

INGREDIENTS

2 cups **raw hazelnuts**

¾ cup **full-fat coconut milk**

½ cup **honey** (or ½ cup + 1 T. pure maple syrup or coconut nectar)

½ cup good quality **cacao powder** (preferably raw, organic)

2 T. each of **virgin coconut oil** and **homemade ghee**, melted (or use ¼ cup of just one)

¾ tsp. pure **vanilla extract**

2-3 pinches **sea salt**

INSTRUCTIONS

1. Preheat oven to 350° F. Roast hazelnuts on a baking sheet in the oven for 10 minutes.
2. Remove hazelnuts from oven and place on a clean, fully dampened tea towel. Wrap the towel around the hot hazelnuts and rub vigorously until all the skins are removed. (It is fine to have a few skins remain on.)
3. Place blanched hazelnuts into food processor with an S-blade and process for a few minutes until mixture becomes creamy. Stop occasionally to scrape down the sides.
4. Then add the rest of the ingredients (coconut milk, sweetener, cacao powder, melted coconut oil and ghee, vanilla and salt). Process until the mixture is creamy and smooth. Again, stop to scrape down the sides as necessary.
5. Pour into mason jars with lids and store in the fridge for up to 2 weeks—if it lasts that long!

Note: Flavour is enhanced when left at room temperature for 30 minutes. If you need it spreadable, leave at room temperature for 30-60 minutes.

TIPS
- *Check honey resource on p. 12 for delicious, mild-tasting, creamy raw honey. It's 100% pure Canadian, well-priced, and they deliver.*

LEMON CURD *made with Honey*

Okay, this is delicious enough to eat with a spoon, but I try to behave and put it in things. Try Lemon Tarts (p.67), Parfait Indulgence (p.54), Mini Chocolate Cups (p.120), or a fruit pizza. Use as a cake filling, or enjoy on pancakes, cookies, muffins, ice cream or oatmeal. Use as a fruit dip for fresh fruit like strawberries and bananas, or fold into coconut whipped cream and make a lemon mousse or ice cream. Be sure to use fresh lemons—bottled lemon juice will not do!

Makes about 1½ cups

INGREDIENTS

1 packed T. **lemon zest** *(approximately 3-4 large lemons)*
⅔ cup **freshly squeezed lemon juice** *(approximately 3-4 large lemons)*
6 **large eggs** total: 5 **yolks** and 1 **whole**
⅓ cup **honey** *(if you prefer sweeter, use extra T.)*
4 tablespoons **grass-fed unsalted butter**, cut into small pieces

INSTRUCTIONS

1. Zest lemons first. Then juice lemons. Set aside.
2. In a medium glass or stainless-steel bowl, whisk together the 5 egg yolks and one whole egg. Add lemon juice and honey and whisk until well combined.
3. Pour mixture into a large saucepan on medium heat, **stirring continuously** with a silicone spatula, until mixture thickens, approximately 5-6 minutes.
4. Remove the bowl from the heat. (Optional: Immediately pour through a fine strainer to remove any lumps. Press through with spatula, if necessary.)
5. Whisk the butter into the mixture until it melts; then whisk in the lemon zest until well-blended.
6. Transfer mixture to a bowl. Cover with a circle of parchment (or plastic wrap), pushing it down to touch the curd. Set aside to cool to room temperature, about 10 minutes. (The curd will thicken as it cools.)
7. Store in sealed jars in fridge for up to 2 weeks, or freezer for up to 6 months.

TIPS

• *Use only freshly squeezed lemon juice.*
• *If you want a smoother version (i.e. without the lemon zest pieces), then in step #2, put lemon zest in with lemon juice and when you press the curd through the mesh strainer (in step #4), zest bits will be removed. Personally, I like the little bits of lemon zest left in.*
• *If you prefer to make this in a bain marie (in a bowl over simmering water—be sure bowl does not touch water)—it will take longer to thicken, about 15-20 minutes.*
• *Check honey resource on p. 12 for delicious, mild-tasting, creamy raw honey. It's 100% pure Canadian, well-priced, and they deliver.*

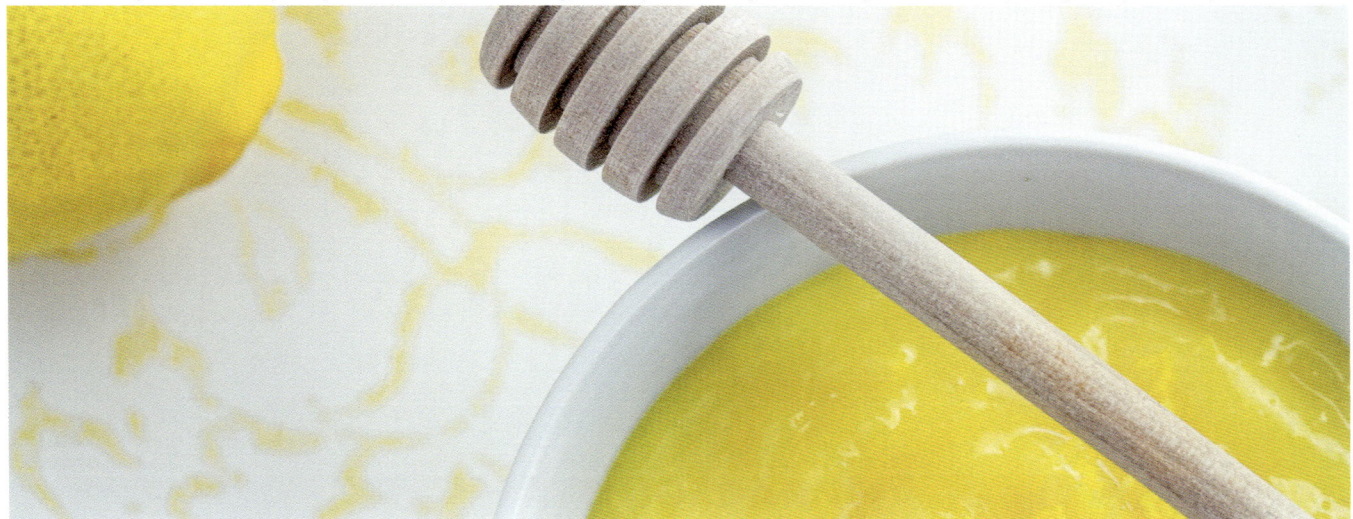

No-Cook FRUIT JAM

GF DF NF EF V P

What do they say? Fresh is best? Well this is fresh jam. This is a fresh tasting jam because it isn't cooked like traditional jam—you really taste the fruit. And the splash of lemon juice just livens up the fruit flavour. This is a quick and easy jam recipe and you can use with almost any fruit. No labour-intensive canning required. Traditional jam also contains a large amount of refined sugar; this contains no added sweetener (adding healthy sweetener is optional). Fresh fruit when it's picked ripe is often sweet enough so be sure to get good quality, local, fresh fruit in season. Make up the size of batch you like to keep fresh in the fridge and freeze the rest. Use in recipes: Banana Sugar-Free Cookies —Thumbprint version (p.29), Parfaits (p.54), on Gluten-Free Banana Muffins (p.96), and of course on toast!

INGREDIENTS

2 cups **fresh or frozen** *(thawed)* **fruit** such as: raspberries, blueberries, strawberries, blackberries, mangos, peaches, apricots, pineapple, kiwi fruit
2 T. **chia seeds**
Optional: Add 1-2 tsp. **fresh lemon juice,** 2 T. **pure maple syrup** and ½ tsp. **vanilla extract.**

INSTRUCTIONS

1. Blend ingredients together in a food processor until well blended.
2. Let sit for 30 minutes or until it thickens.
3. Refrigerate in sealed container such as a mason jar. Keeps for up to 2 weeks in fridge or 6 months in the freezer

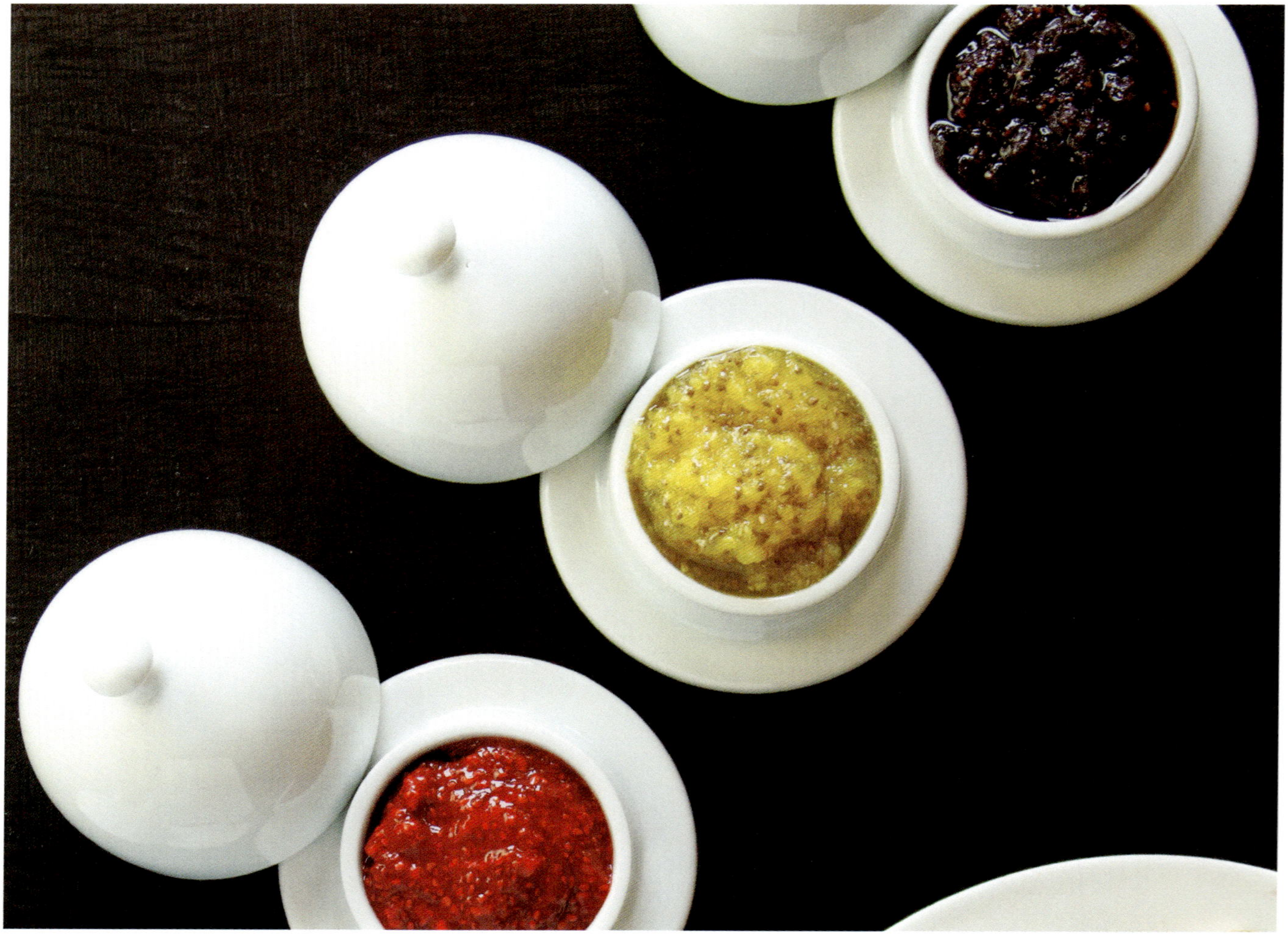

Almond MILK

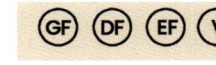

If you've only tasted commercial almond milk, you are in for a treat! This is amazingly fresh tasting and absolutely delicious. Drink it, use it in cereal, smoothies and in recipes that call for alternative milks. The equipment you need for this is a good high-speed blender (such as Blendtec or Vitamix) and a nut-milk bag (which you can buy online or from the health food store). I make these nut milks so often that I bought myself an automatic nut-milk maker—no regrets! However, you can easily make with a nut milk bag by squeezing the milk from the pulp. With this recipe, I also make other plant-based milks (see adaptations below). Be sure to try these homemade milks with Easy Nutty Granola (p.95), Turmeric & Spice Millet Breakfast Bowl (p.94) and Lattés & Frappés (p.98-99).

INGREDIENTS

1½ cups *(approx. 250 g)* **raw, organic, European almonds** *(see Tips)*
5 or 6 cups **water** *(amount of water is flexible, depending on your tastes)*

INSTRUCTIONS

1. Soak almonds in sealed container overnight in fridge.
2. Drain and rinse well.
3. Place all ingredients in high-speed blender (you may need to do in 2 batches to avoid overflow) and blend for approx. 2 minutes.
4. Pour almond milk into a nut milk bag placed over a large bowl or measuring cup.
5. Squeeze milk from bag. This will take 3 or 4 minutes, so be patient. (Save pulp for other uses—see Tips).
6. Almond milk will keep well in a sealed jar in the fridge for 4 or 5 days. Store the rest in the freezer until ready for use. (Just be sure to leave 1-2" space for expansion.)

TIPS
- *I highly recommend organic, European almonds. They have a beautiful almond flavour. However, you can use any raw almonds.*
- *Save almond pulp for use in cookies, crackers, etc. Or dehydrate and use as gluten-free bread crumbs.*

WAYS YOU CAN ADAPT OR ENHANCE THIS RECIPE
- *You can substitute other raw nuts or seeds for the almonds, such as raw cashews, hazelnuts, Brazil nuts, pecans, walnuts, macadamias, pumpkin seeds, sunflower seeds, sesame seeds. Some harder nuts (like hazelnuts and Brazil nuts) may need longer soaking times. (Also see Cashew Milk & Creams, p.148.)*
- *For Sweetened Almond Milk, add to the blender: 5 soft medjool dates, 1½ tsp. pure vanilla extract, pinch sea salt (and even a pinch of cinnamon).*

Cashew MILK & CREAMS

Cashew Milk is the creamiest of the nut milks. All nut milks differ in flavour, texture, body and creaminess. The key to making cashew milk or cream is to use RAW cashews, preferably whole since they are less dry than cashew pieces. They are pretty flavourless on their own (so it's best to add flavoured items to food and beverages). Because of the fat content of cashews, they produce very creamy products! Yum! Cashew cream is a dream vegan-chef staple. It is another substitute for dairy in many ways. It is best to use a highspeed blender, such as a Vitamix or Blendtec to get the best results (creamy and smooth). Use a dollop of the Thick, Sweetened or Strawberry Cashew Creams on Apple Tart Pie (p.47), Pear Crumble (p.59), Banana Cake (p.43), Maple Syrup Pie (p.64), Pumpkin Spice Custard Cups or Pumpkin Pie (p.58), as a layer in a Parfait (p.54), or on whatever you desire! The Pourable Cashew Cream is a great alternative to dairy-cream in coffee. I have also been known to use the Thick Cashew Cream for coffee!

#1 - Cashew Milk – Use Almond Milk recipe (previous page), replacing almonds with raw cashews.
#2 – Pourable Cashew Cream – Pourable cream, used for coffee, lattés and frappés.
#3 – Thick Cashew Cream – Cream that could only be scooped or spooned.
#4 – Sweetened Thick Cashew Cream – Sweetened Thick Cashew Cream used for desserts.
#5 – Strawberry Cashew Cream – Thick Cashew Cream flavoured with fresh strawberries.

CASHEW MILK & CREAM
INGREDIENTS

2 cups **raw cashews** *(preferably whole)*

INSTRUCTIONS

1. **#1 - CASHEW MILK** (makes 4-5 cups): Place cashews in bowl and add enough cold water to cover them by an inch. Let soak for 2 hours or cover and refrigerate overnight. Drain and rinse cashews. Place cashews in high-speed blender and blend until smooth. *(See Tips for more information.)*

2. **#2 - POURABLE CASHEW CREAM** (makes 3½ cups): Follow instructions as for Cashew Milk above, but using less water. Cover cashews in blender with cold water plus a ½ inch. Blend until creamy and smooth. Add water to get desired consistency.

3. **#3 - THICK CASHEW CREAM** (makes 2¼ cups): Follow directions as for Pourable Cashew Cream above, but reduce the amount of water. Start with ¾ cup cold water and add more as needed, to a maximum of 1½ cups. You may have to stop occasionally and scrape sides of blender with spatula.

4. **#4 - SWEETENED CASHEW CREAM** (makes 2¼ cups): Add a small amount of honey, pure maple syrup, coconut nectar or liqueur to Thick Cashew Cream. Note: Reduce the amount of water accordingly.

5. **#5 - "STRAWBERRY CASHEW CREAM"**, omit water and instead blend with 2 cups fresh strawberries, 2 T. tapioca or arrowroot flour and ½ cup honey (or to taste), 2 tsp. vanilla extract, 2 tsp. fresh lemon juice, 2 pinches salt. (This recipe adapted from Sweet Paleo.)

6. Refrigerate for at least 2 hours. Store Cashew Milks and Creams in sealed jars in fridge for up to 5 days. (Or freeze for a few months—be sure to leave a 1-2" space for expansion.)

TIPS
- All creams will thicken up a little after being refrigerated.
- Because there are no emulsifiers or stabilizers as in commercial nut milks, you will need to shake the cashew milk before using.
- Check honey resource on p. 12 for delicious, mild-tasting, creamy raw honey. It's 100% pure Canadian, well-priced, and they deliver.
- If you don't have a high-speed blender, you may have to push your cashew milk or cream through a fine sieve or nut milk bag.

WAYS YOU CAN ADAPT OR ENHANCE THIS RECIPE
- *Add extracts of vanilla, orange, lemon or almond.*
- *Add cinnamon, cardamom, nutmeg, or lavender.*

Oat MILK

A delicious alternative to dairy or nut milk. This recipe produces a milk that is not gelatinous or slimy. Recipe based on "Downshiftology". Serve cold with Easy Nutty Granola (p.95), or any hot or cold cereal. Use in smoothies or baked goods where alternative milks are required. This froths up nicely when steamed to make a beautiful coffee Latté (p.98-99) or a flavoured steamed milk. Delicious used in a Pumpkin Latté (p.98), or my favourite, Caramel Latté (p.98).
Be sure to check out the "Chocolate Milk" and "Strawberry Milk" options below.

Makes about 7 cups

INGREDIENTS

1½ cups **rolled oats** *(preferably organic, gluten-free)*
4 or 5 **digestive enzyme capsules** *(be sure your digestive enzymes contain amylase)*
room temperature **water** *(for soaking)*
4 - 6 cups **ice-cold filtered water** *(see notes in Tips and Adaptations below)*

Sweetened Oat Milk add: *(Optional)*
2 T. **pure maple syrup** *(or 2 medjool dates or healthy sweetener of choice)*
1 tsp. **pure vanilla extract**
pinch **sea salt**

INSTRUCTIONS

1. Place rolled oats in bowl. Empty digestive enzyme capsules into bowl with oats. Cover oats with **room temperature** water plus an extra inch. Stir. Let sit for 15 minutes.
2. Rinse for about 20 seconds, then drain.
3. In a blender or nut milk maker, blend together the **ice-cold filtered water** and the oats. (If choosing to add other ingredients, do before blending.) Blend for 20 seconds. Do not blend for more than 30 seconds—heat can cause it to become gelatinous/slimy.
4. If using a blender, pour milk into nut milk bag to separate the pulp. (Nut milk maker will do this for you.)
5. Pour into jars and refrigerate. This milk with separate because there are no fillers or additives. Simply shake before using.

TIPS
- Using ice cold water and not over-blending are key for a non-gelatinous (non-slimy) product. Some ice cubes can be substituted for water.

WAYS YOU CAN ADAPT OR ENHANCE THIS RECIPE
- If want thicker oat milk simply reduce the amount of ice-cold filtered water to your liking. Some people like to make this recipe with just 3 or 4 cups of water. If you want Oat "Cream", reduce water significantly.
- Variations:
  For "Oat & Hemp Milk", add hemp seeds.
  For "Chocolate Milk", add cacao powder and healthy sweetener.
  For "Strawberry Milk", blend in fresh or frozen strawberries—or berry of choice.

ACKNOWLEDGMENTS

I want to thank my main taster and encourager, my husband, Marc, for your continual love and support. You are the best. I love you and appreciate you.

Thank you, Danic, my cherished son, for being a willing taster and taking my "excess" creations. I appreciate your artistic eye and technical support. You are amazing. I love you forever.

Thank you, Kierra, my book designer, for your extraordinary artistic talents and competence. I love you, my sweet great-niece.

Thank you, Susan E. for being willing to help me with so much of the proofreading and editing — you are so helpful and good at it. I love you, my precious friend.

Thank you, Marcelle, for giving me the nudge to complete this during the 2020/2021 pandemic. I love you like a sister.

Thank you, Susan P. for having a good look at my recipes to make sure there were no mistakes. Your keen eye is appreciated. Baker-buddies forever.

Thank you, cousin Bob, for proofreading the recipes. I like that we share a love of hiking and baking.

Thank you, Lynn, for being a willing proofreader. We will keep walking for chocolate.

Thank you, our dear friends and neighbours, Susan & Tom, for your willingness and enthusiasm to always try my experiments. I love you guys.

I have so much gratitude for all my friends—you have encouraged me to continue and finish this project, and at one time or another you have done some tasting.

Thank you Katherine & Gerhard at Friesens Printers for being so lovely to work with.

And thank you to all those who came before me with great recipes, including a few generations of my family. You have all inspired me.

RECIPE INDEX

BARS
Apple Oat Squares 26
Date Squares 28
Fudgy Butternut Squash Espresso Brownies 77
Lemon Goji Almond Coconut Energy Bars 31
Maple Pecan Bars 31
Orange Fig Bars 28
Peanut Butter Swirl Protein Bars 25
Pecan Rice Crispy Triangles 39
Pistachio Lime Squares 23
Toasted Almonds 'n Honey Rice Crispy Squares 127

BASICS
Almond Milk 147
Blueberry Sauce (cooked & raw versions) 142
Caramel Sauces 131-133
Caramelized Apples 141
Cashew Milk & Cashew Creams 148
Chocolate Sauces, Ganache & Frosting 134-136
Crust: "Graham" Crust 139
Crust: Butter-Vinegar Shortbread Pie Crust 140
Crust: Easy Oil Pie Crust 137
Crust: Pecan Oat Crust 139
Crust: Spelt & Butter Shortbread Crust 138
Date Paste 143
Hazel-Nut-Ella Chocolate Spread (homemade "Nutella") 144
Lemon Curd made with Honey 145
No-Cook Fruit Jam 146
Oat Milk 149
Pecan Praline Butter 143
Raspberry Coulis 142

BEVERAGES
Citrus Martini 101
Ginger & Turmeric Hot Beverage 102
Ginger & Turmeric Iced Frappé 102
Iced Lattés & Frappés 99
Lattés 98-99
Mexican Chili & Cinnamon Hot Chocolate 100
Orange Julia 101

BREAKFASTS
Blackberry & Lemon Clafouti 97
Dutch Apple Pancakes 93
Easy Nutty Granola 95
Gluten-free Banana Muffins 96
Turmeric & Spice Millet Breakfast Bowl 94

CAKES
Banana Cake with Crunchy Topping 43
Blueberry & Vanilla Gluten-Free Coffee Cake 44
Chocolate & Chili Quinoa Cake with Chocolate-Chili Ganache Sauce 81
Flourless Chocolate Cake with Raspberry Coulis 86
Flourless Chocolate Cake with Sugarless Chocolate Frosting 86
Flourless Chocolate Cake with Whiskey Caramel Sauce 86
Queen Elizabeth Date Cake 42
Quinoa Carrot Cake 41

CHEESECAKES
Lemon Cashew Cheesecake 63
Baked Cashew Cheesecake with Caramelized Apples 69
Berrylicious Cashew Cheesecake 49
Lemon & Lime Frozen Mini Cashew Cheesecakes 57

CHOCOLATE
Brown Butter & Rosemary Chocolate Tartlets with Sea Salt 71
Chocolate & Chili Quinoa Cake with Chocolate-Chili Ganache 81
Chocolate Bark with Various Toppings 75
Chocolate Chevre Truffles – 3 Ways 89
Chocolate Chip Cookie Dough in Chocolate Cups 123
Chocolate Espresso Ganache Tart 83
Chocolate Espresso Pâté 82
Chocolate, Oats & Coconut No-Bake Drop Cookies 32
Chocolate Mocha Latté 99
Chocolate Popcorn 124
Chocolate Sauces, Ganache & Frosting 134-136
Coconut Clouds in Dark Chocolate 79
Crunchy Chocolate Bites 91
Dark Chocolate Pecan Clusters with Sea Salt 87
Double Chocolate Fudge Mini Tarts 129
Flourless Chocolate Cake with Raspberry Coulis 86
Flourless Chocolate Cake with Sugarless Chocolate Frosting 86
Flourless Chocolate Cake with Whiskey Caramel Sauce 86
Flourless Chocolate Cupcakes with Sugarless Chocolate Frosting 45
Fudgsicles 107
Fudgy Butternut Squash Espresso Brownies 77
Hazel-Nut-Ella Chocolate Spread (homemade "Nutella") 144
Mexican Chili & Cinnamon Hot Chocolate 100
Mini Chocolate Cups with Various Fillings 120
Nutella Truffles 78
Nutella Chocolate Cups 78
OMG! Chocolate Avocado Puddings 85
Patti's Peppermint Patties 74
Peanut Butter Chocolate Nib'd Truffles 73
Peanut Butter Swirl Protein Bars 25
White Chocolate & Macadamia Tahini Cookies 37

COOKIES
Almond Oatmeal Cookies 36
Almond Shortbread Fingers 33
Banana Oatmeal Sugar-Free Cookies 29
Chocolate, Oats & Coconut No-Bake Drop Cookies 32
Creamy Coconut Superfood Cookies 27
Grandad's Oatmeal Cookies 35
Maple Shortbread 27
White Chocolate & Macadamia Tahini Cookies 37

CRUMBLES & CRISPS
Blueberry Crisp 55
Pear Crumble 59

CRUSTS
Butter-Vinegar Shortbread Pie Crust 140
Easy Oil Pie Crust 137
Graham Crust 139
Pecan Oat Crust 139
Spelt & Butter Shortbread Crust 138

CUPCAKES
Flourless Chocolate Cupcakes with Sugarless Chocolate Frosting 45

CUSTARDS
Baked Coconut Eggnog Custard 51
Lemon Curd made with Honey 145
Pumpkin Spice Custard Cups 58
Vanilla & Lemon Custard Fruit Dip 113

FROZEN DESSERTS & TREATS
Banana Soft Serve Ice Cream 121
Berrylicious Cashew Cheesecake 49
Blueberry "Instant" Ice Cream 50
Fudgsicles 107
Ginger & Turmeric Iced Frappé 102
Iced Lattés & Frappés 99
Lemon & Lime Frozen Mini Cashew Cheesecakes 57
Orange Creamsicles 109

KIDS (see also 'Snacks')
"Just for Kids" Recipes & Recipe Ideas 116-117
Banana Soft Serve Ice Cream 121
Chocolate Chip Cookie Dough in Chocolate Cups 123
Chocolate Popcorn 124
Double Chocolate Fudge Mini Tarts 129
Fruit on a Stick 119
Mini Chocolate Cups with Various Fillings 120
Sprinkles 125
Toasted Almonds 'n Honey Rice Crispy Squares 127

MUFFINS
Gluten-free Banana Muffins 96

PARFAITS
Parfait Indulgence 54

PIES
Apple Tart Pie with Butter Crust 47
Fresh Raspberry Pie with Raspberry-Honey Glaze 53
Maple Syrup Pie 64
Pumpkin Pie 58

PLANT-BASED MILKS
Almond Milk 147
Cashew Milk & Cashew Creams 148
Oat Milk 149

PUDDINGS
Coconut Chia Pudding with Berry Sauce 61
OMG! Chocolate Avocado Puddings 85

SAUCES
Blueberry Sauce 142
Caramel Sauces 131-133
Chocolate Sauces, Ganache & Frosting 134-136
Raspberry Coulis 142

SNACKS (see also 'Kids')
Apple Chips 110
Candied Maple Walnuts 108
Candied Maple Pumpkin Seeds 108
Caramel Corn with Macadamia Nuts 104
Chocolate Popcorn 124
Fruit on a Stick 119
Fudgsicles 107
Honey Butter Coconut Chips & 3-Seed Coconut Clusters 105
Orange Creamsicles 109
Power Balls 109
Salty, Sweet & Spicy Maple Pecans 114
Vanilla & Lemon Custard Fruit Dip 113

SPREADS
Chocolate Espresso Pâté 82
Date Paste 143
Hazel-Nut-Ella Chocolate Spread (Nutella) 144
Lemon Curd made with Honey 145
No-Cook Fruit Jam 146
Pecan Praline Butter 143

TARTS
Apple Tart Pie with Butter Crust 47
Brown Butter & Rosemary Chocolate Tartlets with Sea Salt 71
Caramel Pecan Banana Tarts 65
Chocolate Espresso Ganache Tart 83
Double Chocolate Fudge Mini Tarts 129
Lemon Tarts 67